Benign and Malignant Tumours

DEDICATION

We dedicate this book to the Organizing Committee: E. Johannison, P. Melzer, H.S. Jacobs, P.C. Sizonenko, F.H. Schroder and F. Comite and to all our colleagues whose work with GnRH analogues is increasing the quality of life for individuals suffering the wide range of medical conditions benefited by the use of these agents.

B. H. Vickery
B. Lunenfeld

VOLUME III

Benign and Malignant Tumours

GnRH ANALOGUES
IN CANCER AND
HUMAN
REPRODUCTION

Edited by
B. H. Vickery and B. Lunenfeld

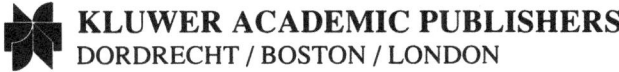
KLUWER ACADEMIC PUBLISHERS
DORDRECHT / BOSTON / LONDON

Distributors

for the United States and Canada: Kluwer Academic Publishers, PO Box 358,
Accord Station, Hingham, MA 02018-0358, USA
for all other countries: Kluwer Academic Publishers Group, Distribution Center,
PO Box 322, 3300 AH Dordrecht, The Netherlands

British Library Cataloguing in Publication Data

GnRH analogues in cancer and human reproduction.
   Vol.3. Benign and malignant tumours.
   1. Women. Reproductive system. Cancer. Drug therapy
   I. Vickery, B. H. (Brian H.), *1941–*   II. Lunenfeld, Bruno
   616.99'465061

ISBN-13: 978-94-010-6810-9   e-ISBN-13: 978-94-009-0723-2
DOI: 10.1007/978-94-009-0723-2

Library of Congress Cataloging-in-Publication Data

GnRH analogues in cancer and human reproduction / edited by B.H. Vickery and B. Lunenfeld
     p.   cm.
   Includes bibliographical references.
   Contents: Vol. 1. Basic aspects – v. 2. GnRH analogues in reproduction and gynecology – v. 3.
Benign and malignant tumours – v. 4. Precocious puberty, contraception, safety issues.

    1. Generative organs – – Diseases – – Hormone therapy – – Congresses. 2. Luteinizing hormone
releasing hormone – – Derivatives – – Therapeutic use – – Congresses. 3. Generative
organs – – Cancer – – Hormone therapy – – Congresses. I. Vickery, Brian H., 1941 –   . II. Lunenfeld,
Bruno.
   [DNLM: 1. Neoplasms – – drug therapy. 2. Pituitary Hormone Releasing Hormones – – physiology. 3.
Reproduction – – drug effects. WK 515 G572]
   RC877.G57 1989
   618'.0461 – – dc20
   DNLM/DLC
   for Library of Congress   89-24592
                                               CIP

Copyright

Published in the United Kingdom by Kluwer Academic Publishers, PO Box 55,
Lancaster, UK.

Kluwer Academic Publishers BV incorporates the publishing programmes of D. Reidel,
Martinus Nijhoff, Dr W. Junk and MTP Press.

CONTENTS

CONTENTS OF OTHER VOLUMES

Volume II. GnRH Analogues in Reproduction and Gynecology

Volume IV. Precocious Puberty, Contraception, Safety Issues

PREFACE

These four volumes comprising "GnRH Analogues in Cancer and Human
Reproduction" are a distillation of the presentations of the
invited speakers at a landmark International Symposium bearing the
same name, organized by one of us (B.L.) and held in Geneva,
Switzerland in February 1988. The Symposium was truly
interdisciplinary spanning gonadal hormone dependent disease
including various forms of cancer and ranging to control of
fertility, both pro- and conception. The international flavor can
be caught from the 480 participants and 259 contributors drawn
from 14 countries. The Symposium, and therefore this book, would
not have been possible without the backing of The International
Committee for Research in Reproduction and the sponsorship of the
International Society of Gynecologic Endocrinology, The Swiss
Society of Fertility and Sterility, The University of Geneva
School of Medicine, The Swiss Society of Endocrinology and The US
Foundation for Studies in Reproduction Inc., and help from the
World Health Organization.

B. H. Vickery
B. Lunenfeld
June 1989

LIST OF CONTRIBUTORS
TO THE SERIES

A. Abbondante
First Institute of Obstetrics and
    Gynecology
University "La Sapienza"
Rome, Italy

P. Abel
Department of Urology
Hammersmith Hospital
DuCane Road
London W12 OHS, UK

H. Abramovici
Departments of Obstetrics and
    Gynecology
Rambam Medical Center and Carmel
    Hospital, Technion
Israel Institute of Technology
Haifa 31096, Israel

V. Aleandri
First Institute of Obstetrics and
    Gynecology
University "La Sapienza"
Rome, Italy

Michel L. Aubert
Department of Pediatrics and Genetics
Division of Biology of Growth and
    Reproduction
University of Geneva Medical School
1211 Geneva 4, Switzerland

Tom M. Badger
Reproductive Endocrine Unit
Vincent Memorial Research Laboratories
Boston, MA 02114, USA

Sandor Bajusz
Veterans Administration Medical Center
1601 Perdido Street
New Orleans, LA 71046, USA

P. Barriere
IVF Department
CHU Nantes
44035-Nantes Cedex 01, France

H. Bartermann
Urologische Universitatsklinik Kiel
Arnold-Heller Strasse 7
D-2300 Kiel 1, FRG

M. Bartholomew
Department of Medicine/Endocrinology
Milton S. Hershey Medical Center
Pennsylvania State University
PO Box 850, Hershey, PA 17033, USA

D. Beck
Departments of Obstetrics and
    Gynecology
Ramban Medical Center and Carmel
    Hospital, Technion
Israel Institute of Technology
Haifa 31096, Israel

G. Benagiano
First Institute of Obstetrics and
    Gynecology
University "La Sapienza"
Rome, Italy

G. Bender
Department of Obstetrics and Gynecology
Staedtische Kliniken
Grafenstrasse 9
D-6100 Darmstadt, FRG

Z. Ben-Rafael
Interdepartmental Unit of Human
    Reproduction
Department of Obstetrics and Gynecology
The Chaim Sheba Medical Center and
    Sackler School of Medicine
Tel-Hashomer 52621, Israel

M. Berezin
Institute of Endocrinology
The Chaim Sheba Medical Center
Tel-Hashomer 52621, Israel

G. Bettendorf
UKE Frauenklinik
Division of Endocrinology
Martinistrasse 52
2000 Hamburg 20, FRG

Zvi Binor
Section of Reproductive
   Endocrinology/Infertility
Department of Obstetrics and Gynecology
Rush Medical College
Chicago, IL 60612, USA

W.P. Black
University Department of Obstetrics and
   Gynaecology
Glasgow Royal Infirmary
Glasgow G31 2ER, UK

J. Blankstein
Interdepartmental Unit of Human
   Reproduction
Department of Obstetrics and Gynecology
The Chaim Sheba Medical Center and
   Sackler School of Medicine
Tel-Hashomer 52621, Israel

Robert M. Blizzard
Department of Pediatrics
University of Virginia Medical School
PO Box 386
Charlottesville, VA 22901, USA

Zeev Blumenfeld
Departments of Obstetrics and
   Gynecology
Ramban Medical Center and Carmel
   Hospital
Technion, Israel Institute of Technology
Haifa 31096, Israèl

Paul A. Boepple
Reproductive Endocrine Unit
Massachusetts General Hospital
Rear Blossom Street
Boston, MA 02114, USA

L. Boubli
Gynecologie-Obstetrique
Hopital Michel Levy, Annexe Conception
84a Rue de Lodi
13281 Marseille Cedex 6, France

A. Boucher
Department of Medicine/Endocrinology
Milton S. Hershey Medical Center
Pennsylvania State University
PO Box 850, Hershey, PA 17033, USA

Cyril Bowers
Endocrine Unit
Tulane University School of Medicine
New Orleans, LA 70112, USA

W. Braendel
UKE Frauenklinik
Division of Endocrinology
Martinistrasse 52
2000 Hamburg 20, FRG

J.M. Brandes
Departments of Obstetrics and
   Gynecology
Ramban Medical Center and Carmel
   Hospital, Technion
Israel Institute of Technology
Haifa 31096, Israel

R. Brauner
Unit of Pediatric Endocrinology and
   Diabetes
Hospital des Enfants Malades
75015 Paris, France

M. Breckwoldt
Department of Obstetrics and Gynecology
Division of Clinical Endocrinology
University of Freiburg
D-7800 Freiburg-im-Breisgau, FRG

Th. Bremen
Department of Obstetrics and Gynecology
Staedtische Kliniken
Grafenstrasse 9
D-6100 Darmstadt, FRG

Todd D. Brodie
Reproductive Endocrine Unit
Vincent Memorial Research Laboratories
Boston, MA 02114, USA

I.A. Brosens
Laboratory for Gynaecological
   Physiopathology
UZ Gasthuisberg
KU Leuven, Belgium

Robert Browneller
Abbott Laboratories
Abbott Park, IL 60064, USA

S.K. Burt
Pharmaceutical Discovery Division
Abbott Laboratories
Abbott Park, IL 60064, USA

Eugene N. Bush
Pharmaceutical Discovery Division
Abbott Laboratories
Abbott Park, IL 60064, USA

M. Camus
Center for Reproductive Medicine
Medical Campus, Vrije University Brussel
Laarbeeklaan 101
1090 Brussels, Belgium

R.J. Capetola
Ortho Pharmaceutical Corporation
Route 202
Raritan, NJ 08869, USA

R. Caplan
Department of Medicine/Endocrinology
Milton S. Hershey Medical Center
Pennsylvanian State University
PO Box 850, Hershey, PA 71033, USA

M. Carter
University Department of Obstetrics and
    Gynaecology
Glasgow Royal Infirmary
Glasgow G31 2ER, UK

E. Caspi
Department of Obstetrics and Gynecology
Assaf Harofe Medical Center
Zerefin, Israel

B. Charbonnel
IVF Department
CHU Nantes
44035-Nantes Cedex 01, France

J.L. Chaussain
Foundation de Recherche en
    Homonologie
PB110
94268 Fresnes Cedex, France

Claudia Chillik
Department of Obstetrics and Gynecology
Eastern Virginia Medical School
Norfolk, VA 23507, USA

Jean Cohen
Clinique Marignan
3 rue Marignan
75008 Paris, France

Ana Maria Comaru-Schally
Veterans Administration Medical Center
1601 Perdido Street
New Orleans, LA 70146, USA

Florence Comite
Department of Medicine and Gynecology
Yale University School of Medicine
New Haven, CT 06510-8063, USA

C. Conaghan
University Department of Obstetrics and
    Gynaecology
Glasgow Royal Infirmary
Glasgow G31 2ER, UK

P. Michael Conn
Department of Pharmacology
University of Iowa College of Medicine
Iowa City, IO 52242, USA

Angelo Conti
Ch. de Mornex 6
1003 Lausanne, Switzerland

F. Cornillie
Laboratory for Gynaecological
    Pathophysiology
UZ Gasthuisberg
KU Leuven, Belgium

R.M. Couch
Department of Pediatrics and Pathology
University of British Columbia
BC's Children's Hospital
Vancouver, BC V6H 3V4, Canada

J.R.T. Coutts
University Department of Obstetrics and
    Gynaecology
Glasgow Royal Infirmary
Glasgow G31 2ER, UK

J. Cox
Department of Urology
Central Middlesex Hospital
London, UK

John D. Crawford
Children's Service
Massachusetts General Hospital
Fruit Street
Boston, MA 02114, USA

John F. Crigler, Jr.
Department of Medicine
Division of Endocrinology, Children's
     Hospital
300 Longwood Avenue
Boston, MA 02115, USA

William F. Crowley Jr.
Departments of Medicine and Gynecology
Massachusetts General Hospital
Boston, MA 02114, USA

Lionel Cusan
Department of Molecular Endocrinology
Laval University Medical Center
Quebec G1V 4G2, Canada

Douglas R. Danforth
Department of Obstetrics and Gynecology
Eastern University Medical School
Norfolk, VA 23507, USA

F. Calais da Silva
A.Z. Middelheim
Antwerp 2020, Belgium

Adi Davidson
Interdepartmental Unit of Human
     Reproduction
Department of Obstetrics and Gynecology
The Chaim Sheba Medical Center and
     Sackler School of Medicine
Tel-Hashomer 52621, Israel

R. Deghenghi
Debiopharm SA
1003 Lausanne, Switzerland

F.H. de Jong
Department of Medicine II and Clinical
     Endocrinology
Erasmus University
Rotterdam, The Netherlands

L. Denis
A.Z. Middelheim
Antwerp 2020, Belgium

M. De Pauw
A.Z. Middelheim
Antwerp 2020, Belgium

J. De Schacht
Center for Reproductive Medicine
Medical Campus, Vrije Universiteit Brussel
Laarbeeklaan 101
1090 Brussels, Belgium

P. Devroey
Center for Reproductive Medicine
Medical Campus, Vrije Universiteit Brussel
Laarbeeklaan 101
1090 Brussels, Belgium

Gilbert Diaz
Pharmaceutical Discovery Division
Abbott Laboratories
Abbott Park, IL 60064, USA

M. Dirnfeld
Departments of Obstetrics and
     Gynecology
Ramban Medical Center and Carmel
     Hospital, Technion
Israel Institute of Technology
Haifa 31096, Israel

W. Paul Dmowski
Section of Reproductive
     Endocrinology/Infertility
Department of Obstetrics and Gynecology
Rush Medical College
Chicago, IL 60612, USA

Joshua Dor
Interdepartmental Unit of Human
     Reproduction
Department of Obstetrics and Gynecology
The Chaim Sheba Medical Center and
     Sackler School of Medicine
Tel-Hashomer 52621, Israel

J. Drago
Department of Medicine/Endocrinology
Milton S. Hershey Medical Center
Pennsylvania State University
PO Box 850, Hershey, PA 17033, USA

S.L.S. Drop
Sophia Children's Hospital
160 Gordelweg
3038 GE Rotterdam, The Netherlands

André Dupont
Department of Molecular Endocrinology
Laval University Medical Center
Quebec G1V 4G2, Canada

Anand S. Dutta
Pharmaceutical Division
Imperial Chemical Industries plc
Mereside, Alderley Park
Macclesfield, Cheshire SK10 4TG, UK

L. Edwards
Westminster Hospital
London SW1 2AP, UK

Adreian Elenbogen
Interdepartmental Unit of Human
    Reproduction
Department of Obstetrics and Gynecology
The Chaim Sheba Medical Center and
    Sackler School of Medicine
Tel-Hashomer 52621, Israel

D. Elia
Clinique Marignan
3 rue Marignan
75008 Paris, France

Jean Emond
Laval University Medical Center
Quebec G1V 4G2, Canada

G. Emons
Klinik für Franenheilkunde und
    Geburtshilfe
Institute für Biochemische Endokrinologie
Medizurische Universiteit zu Lübeck
D-2400 Lübeck, FRG

K. Engelbart
Hoechst AG
D-6230 Frankfurt 80, FRG

R. Erny
Gynecologie-Obstetrique
Hospital Michael Levy, Annexe Conception
84a rue de Lodi
13281 Marseille Cedex 6, France

N. Farah
Department of Urology
Central Middlesex Hospital
London, UK

S. Finnie
University Department of Obstetrics and
    Gynaecology
Glasgow Royal Infirmary
Glasgow G31 2ER, UK

J. Fleming
Department of Urology
Central Middlesex Hospital
London, UK

R. Fleming
University Department of Obstetrics and
    Gynaecology
Glasgow Royal Infirmary
Glasgow G31 2ER, UK

J.A. Foekens
Division of Endocrine Oncology
Rotterdam Cancer Institute
The Dr. Daniel den Hoed Cancer Center,
    Groene Hilledijk 301
3075 EA Rotterdam, The Netherlands

I. Fogelman
Department of Nuclear Medicine
Guy's Hospital
London, UK

Karl Folkers
Institute for Biomedical Research
The University of Texas at Austin
Austin, TX 78712, USA

C. Fouprie
Foundation de Recherche en
    Hormonologie
PB110
94268 Fresnes Cedex, France

R. Francois
Foundation de Recherche en
    Hormonologie
PB110
94268 Fresnes Cedex, France

Andrew J. Friedman
Brigham and Women's Hospital
Fertility and Endocrine Unit
75 Francis Street
Boston, MA 02115, USA

Barrington J.A. Furr
Bioscience I. Department
ICI Pharmaceuticals plc
Alderley Park, Macclesfield
Cheshire SK10 4TG, UK

F. Geisthövel
Department of Obstetrics and Gynecology
Division of Clinical Endocrinology
University of Freiburg
D-7800 Freiburg-im-Breisgau, FRG

B. Gilks
Department of Pediatrics and Pathology
University of British Columbia
BC's Children's Hospital
Vancouver BC V6H 3V4, Canada

L. Giode
Department of Medicine/Endocrinology
Milton S. Hershey Medical Center
Pennsylvania State University
PO Box 850, Hershey, PA 17033, USA

A. Golan
Department of Obstetrics and Gynecology
Assaf Harofe Medical Center
Zerefin, Israel

Jessie C. Goodpasture
Institute of Biological Sciences
Syntex Research
3401 Hillview Avenue
Palo Alto, CA 94304, USA

R. Gordon
Department of Medicine/Endocrinology
Milton S. Hershey Medical Center
Pennsylvania State University
PO Box 850, Hershey, PA 17033, USA

Jonathan Greer
Pharmaceutical Discovery Division
Abbott Laboratories
Abbott Park, IL 60064, USA

Melvin M. Grumbach
Department of Pediatrics
University of California San Francisco
San Francisco, CA 94943, USA

F. Hadziselimovic
Children's Hospital Basle
Römergasse 8
CH-4005 Basle, Switzerland

D.W. Hahn
Ortho Pharmaceutical Corporation
Route 202
Raritan, NJ 08869, USA

M. Hahn
Hoechst AG
D-6230 Frankfurt 80, FRG

H. Halkin
Institute of Endocrinology
The Chaim Sheba Medical Center
Tel-Hashomer 52621, Israel

Janet E. Hall
Reproductive Endocrine Unit
Vincent Memorial Research Laboratories
Boston, MA 02114, USA

M.P.R. Hamilton
University Department of Obstetrics and
 Gynaecology
Glasgow Royal Infirmary
Glasgow G31 2ER, UK

H. Harvey
Department of Medicine/Endocrinology
Milton S. Hershey Medical Center
Pennsylvania State University
PO Box 850, Hershey, PA 17033, USA

Fortuna Haviv
Pharmaceutical Discovery Division
Abbott Laboratories
Abbott Park, IL 60064, USA

M.J. Haxton
University Department of Obstetrics and
 Gynaecology
Glasgow Royal Infirmary
Glasgow G31 2ER, UK

D.L. Healey
Medical Research Center
Monash Medical Center
Prince Henry's Hospital Campus
Melbourne, Australia

A. Herman
Department of Obstetrics and Gynecology
Assaf Harofe Medical Center
Zerefin, Israel

P. Heuschen
Department of Obstetrics and Gynecology
Staedtische Kliniken
Grafenstrasse 9
D-6100 Darmstadt, FRG

P.C. Ho
Department of Obstetrics and Gynecology
University of Hong Kong
Hong Kong

Gary D. Hodgen
Jones Institute for Reproductive Medicine
Eastern University Medical School
Norfolk, VA 23507, USA

J.C. Huber
1st Department of Gynecology and
    Obstetrics
A-1090 Vienna, Austria

Magdalen E. Hull
Division of Reproductive Endocrinology
Department of Obstetrics and Gynecology
State University of New York at Stony
    Brook School of Medicine
Stony Brook, NY 11794-8091, USA

R. Hummelink
Sophia Children's Hospital
160 Gordelweg
3038 GE Rotterdam, The Netherlands

F.G. Hutchinson
Pharmaceutical Department, ICI
    Pharmaceutical plc
Alderley Park, Macclesfield
Cheshire SK10 4TG, UK

Vaclav Insler
Endocrinology Laboratory, Soroka
    Medical Center and
Division of Obstetrics and Gynecology
Clinical Biochemistry Unit, Faculty of
    Health Sciences
Ben-Gurion University of the Negev
Beer-Sheba 84101, Israel

Joseph Itskovitz
Department of Obstetrics and Gynecology
Eastern University Medical School
Norfolk, VA 23507, USA

M.E. Jamieson
University Department of Obstetrics and
    Gynaecology
Glasgow Royal Infirmary
Glasgow G31 2ER, UK

G. Jerabek-Sandow
Hoechst AG
D-6230 Frankfurt 80, FRG

Edwin S. Johnson
Pharmaceutical Discovery Division
Abbott Laboratories
Abbott Park, IL 60064, USA

W. Jäger
Department of Gynecology and Obstetrics
University of Erlangen-Nürnberg
8520 Erlangen, FRG

Themis Kamilaris
Division of Endocrinology
Vanderbilt University School of Medicine
Nashville, TN 37232, USA

Selna L. Kaplan
Department of Pediatrics
University of California San Francisco
San Francisco, CA 94943, USA

R. Kauli
Institute of Pediatric and Adolescent
    Endocrinology
Sackler Faculty of Medicine
Tel Aviv University
Tel Aviv, Israel

Daniel Kenigsberg
Division of Reproductive Endocrinology
Department of Obstetrics and Gynecology
State University of New York at Stony
    Brook School of Medicine
Stony Brook, NY 11794-8091, USA

F. Keuppens
A.Z. Middelheim
Antwerp 2020, Belgium

I. Khan
Center for Reproductive Medicine
Medical Campus, Vrije Universitiet Brussel
Laarbeeklaan 101
1090 Brussels, Belgium

Ludwig Kiesel
Division of Gynecological Endocrinology
Department of Obstetrics and Gynecology
University of Heidelberg
D-6900 Heidelberg, FRG

S. Kille
Hoechst AG
D-6230 Frankfurt 80, FRG

H. Kitson
Department of Pediatrics and Pathology
University of British Columbia
BC's Children's Hospital
Vancouver BC V6H 3V4, Canada

Jan G.M. Klijn
Division of Endocrine Oncology
Rotterdam Cancer Institute
The Dr. Daniel den Hoed Cancer Center,
    Groene Hilledijk 301
3075 EA Rotterdam, The Netherlands

Jasna Knezvic
Department of Pediatrics
University of California San Francisco
San Francisco, CA 94943, USA

R. Knuppen
Klinik für Biochemische Endokrinologie
Medizurische Universiteit zu Lübeck
D-2400 Lübeck, FRG

B. Krauss
Hoechst AG
D-6230 Frankfurt 80, FRG

Renee Kreuter
Department of Pediatrics and Genetics
Division of Biology of Growth and
    Reproduction
University of Geneva Medical School
1211 Geneva 4, Switzerland

Fernand Labrie
Department of Molecular Endocrinology
Laval University Medical Center
Quebec G1V 4G2, Canada

Yves Lacourciere
Laval University Medical Center
Quebec G1V 4G2, Canada

N. Lahlou
Foundation de Recherche en
    Hormonologie
PB110
94268 Fresnes Cedex, France

N. Lang
Department of Gynecology and Obstetrics
University of Erlangen-Nürnberg
8520 Erlangen, FRG

Zvi Laron
Beilinson Medical Center
Petah Tikva 49100, Israel

André Lemay
Endocrinology of Reproduction
Hospital Saint-Francoise D'Asise
Quebec G1L 3L5, Canada

David Levran
Interdepartmental Unit of Human
    Reproduction
Department of Obstetrics and Gynecology
The Chaim Sheba Medical Center and
    Sackler School of Medicine
Tel-Hashomer 52621, Israel

Joseph Levy
Endocrinology Laboratory, Soroka
    Medical Center and
Division of Obstetrics and Gynecology
Clinical Biochemistry Unit, Faculty of
    Health Sciences
Ben-Gurion University of the Negev
Beer-Sheba 84101, Israel

L. Levy
Tel Aviv University
Sackler School of Medicine
Tel Aviv, Israel

G. Leyendecker
Department of Obstetrics and Gynecology
Staedtische Kliniken, Grafenstrasse 9
D-6100 Darmstadt, FRG

D.F.H. Li
Department of Obstetrics and Gynecology
University of Hong Kong
Hong Kong

V. Lichtenburg
UKE Frauenklinik
Division of Endocrinology
Martinistrasse 52
2000 Hamburg 20, FRG

S.L. Lightman
Charing Cross and Westminster Medical
    School
London, UK

Ch. Lindner
UKE Frauenklinik
Division of Endocrinology
Martinistrasse 52
2000 Hamburg 20, FRG

Kathleen Link
Department of Medicine and Pediatrics
Harvard Medical School
Boston, MA 02115, USA

Schlomo Lipitz
Interdepartmental Unit of Human
    Reproduction
Department of Obstetrics and Gynecology
The Chaim Sheba Medical Center and
    Sackler School of Medicine
Tel-Hashomer 52621, Israel

A. Lipton
Department of Medicine/Endocrinology
Milton S. Hershey Medical Center
Pennsylvania State University
PO Box 850, Hershey, PA 17033, USA

P. Lopes
IVF Department
CHU Nantes
44035-Nantes Cedex 01, France

M. Luckhardt
UKE Frauenklinik
Division of Endocrinology
Martinistrasse 52
2000 Hamburg 20, FRG

Bruno Lunenfeld
Institute of Endocrinology
Sheba Medical Center and Bar Ilan
    University
Remat Gan 52621, Israel

E. Lunenfeld
Division of Obstetrics and Gynecology
Soroka Medical Center and Ben-Gurion
    University of the Negev
Beer-Sheba, Israel

J.L. McGuire
Ortho Pharmaceutical Corporation
Route 202
Raritan, NJ 08869, USA

Georgia I. McRae
Institute of Biological Sciences
Syntex Research
Palo Alto, CA 94304, USA

Gilles Manhes
Laval University Medical Center
Quebec G1V 4G2, Canada

Andrea Manni
Department of Medicine/Endocrinology
The Milton S. Hershey Medical Center
The Pennsylvania State University
PO Box 850, Hershey, PA 17033, USA

Joan Mansfield
Reproductive Endocrine Unit
Massachusetts General Hospital
Rear Blossom Street
Boston, MA 02114, USA

Shlomo Maschiach
Interdepartmental Unit of Human
    Reproduction
Department of Obstetrics and Gynecology
The Chaim Sheba Medical Center and
    Sackler School of Medicine
Tel-Hashomer 52621, Israel

W.H.M. Matta
Academic Department of Obstetrics and
    Gynaecology
Royal Free Hospital
London NW3 2QG, UK

Devorah T. Max
Abbott Laboratories
Abbott Park, IL 60064, USA

P. Merat
Pharmaceutical Division
Hoechst Canada Inc.
4045 Cote Vertu
Montreal, Quebec H4R 1R6, Canada

L. Mettler
Department of Obstetrics and Gynecology
University of Kiel
2300 Kiel, FRG

E. Milliet
Gynecologie-Obstetrique
Hopital Michael Levy, Annexe Conception
84a rue de Lodi
13281 Marseille Cedex 6, France

H.W. Minne
Department of Internal Medicine
University of Heidelberg
Heidelberg, FRG

Gerard Monfette
Laval University Medical Center
Quebec G1V 4G2, Canada

A. Morini
First Institute of Obstetrics and
    Gynecology
University "La Sapienza"
Rome, Italy

H. Nachum
Department of Obstetrics and Gynecology
Assaf Harofe Medical Center
Zerefin, Israel

John J. Nestor Jr.
Institute of Bio-Organic Chemistry
Syntex Research
3401 Hillview Avenue
Palo Alto, CA 94304, USA

J. Neulen
Department of Obstetrics and Gynecology
Division of Clinical Endocrinology
University of Freiburg
D-7800 Freiburg-im-Breisgau, FRG

D. Newling
A.Z. Middelheim
Antwerp 2020, Belgium

Eberhard Nieschlag
Max Planck Clinical Research Unit for
    Reproductive Medicine
Institute of Reproductive Medicine of the
    University
D-4400 Münster, FRG

F. Oberheuser
Klinik für Franenheilkunde und
    Geburtshilfe
Institute für Biochemische Endokrinologie
Medizinische Universiteit zu Lübeck
D-2400 Lübeck, FRG

A.J.H. Odink
Sophia Children's Hospital
160 Gordelweg
3038 GE Rotterdam, The Netherlands

E.P.N. O'Donohue
Department of Urology
Central Middlesex Hospital
London, UK

P. Onegana
A.Z. Middelheim
Antwerp 2020, Belgium

W. Oostdijk
Sophia Children's Hospital
160 Gordelweg
3038 GE Rotterdam, The Netherlands

G.S. Pahwa
Klinik für Franenheilkunde und
    Gerburtshilfe
Institute für Biochemische Endokrinologie
Medizinische Universiteit zu Lübeck
D-2400 Lübeck, FRG

Christopher A. Palabrica
Pharmaceutical Discovery Division
Abbott Laboratories
Abbott Park, IL 60064, USA

I. Papadopoulos
Urologische Universitatsklinik Kiel
Arnold-Heller Strasse 7
D-2300 Kiel 1, FRG

H. Parmar
Department of Oncology
Westminster Hospital
London SW1 2AP, UK

C.J. Partsch
Sophia Children's Hospital
160 Gordelweg
3038 GE Rotterdam, The Netherlands

Spyros N. Pavlou
Division of Endocrinology
Vanderbilt University School of Medicine
Nashville, TN 37232, USA

Peg Pepping
Section of Reproductive
    Endocrinology/Infertility
Department of Obstetrics and Gynecology
Rush Medical Center
Chicago, IL 60612, USA

A. Phillips
Ortho Pharmaceutical Corporation
Route 202
Raritan, NJ 08869, USA

R.H. Phillips
Westminster Hospital
London SW1 2AP, UK

F. Piccinno
First Institute of Obstetrics and
    Gynecology
University "La Sapienza"
Rome, Italy

G. Potashnik
Division of Obstetrics and Gynecology
Soroka Medical Center and Ben Gurion
    University of the Negev
Beer Sheba, Israel

P. Puttemans
Laboratory for Gynaecological
    Pathophysiology
Gasthuisberg
KU Leuven, Belgium

Ewa Radwanska
Section of Reproductive
    Endocrinology/Infertility
Department of Obstetrics and Gynecology
Rush Medical College
Chicago, IL 60612, USA

R. Rappaport
Unit of Pediatric Endocrinology and
    Diabetes
Hospital des Enfants Malades
75015 Paris, France

Tommie W. Redding
Veterans Administration Medical Center
1601 Perdido Street
New Orleans, LA 71046, USA

D.M. Ritchie
Ortho Pharmaceutical Corporation
Route 202
Raritan, NJ 08869, USA

Jean Rivier
Salk Institute for Biological Studies
La Jolla, CA 92037, USA

A. Rodin
Department of Gynaecology
Guy's Hospital
London, UK

M. Roger
Foundation de Recherche en
    Hormonologie
PB110
94268 Fresnes Cedex, France

T. Rohner
Department of Medicine/Endocrinology
Milton S. Hershey Medical Center
Pennsylvania State University
PO Box 850, Hershey, PA 17033, USA

R. Ron-El
Department of Obstetrics and Gynecology
Assaf Harofe Medical Center
Zerefin, Israel

Edwina Rudak
Interdepartmental Unit of Human
    Reproduction
Department of Obstetrics and Gynecology
The Chaim Sheba Medical Center and
    Sackler School of Medicine
Tel-Hashomer 52621, Israel

Benno Runnebaum
Division of Gynecological Endocrinology
Department of Obstetrics and Gynecology
University of Heidelberg
D-6900 Heidelberg, FRG

D. Sala
First Institute of Obstetrics and
    Gynecology
Rome, Italy

Lynda M. Sanders
Institute of Pharmaceutical Sciences
Syntex Research
Palo Alto, CA 94304, USA

Jurgen Sandow
Department of Pharmacology
Hoechst AG
D-6230 Frankfurt 80, FRG

R. Santen
Department of Medicine/Endocrinology
Milton S. Hershey Medical Center
Pennsylvania State University
PO Box 850, Hershey, PA 17033, USA

Carlos A. Schaffenburg
5480 Wisconsin Avenue 1014
Chevy Chase, MD 20815, USA

Andrew V. Schally
Endocrine Polypeptide and Cancer
    Institute
Veterans Admininstration Medical Center
    and Section of Experimental Medicine
Department of Medicine, Tulane University
    School of Medicine
New Orleans, LA 70146, USA

S.H. Scharla
Department of Internal Medicine
University of Heidelberg
Heidelberg, FRG

F. Schaumkell
Urologische Universitatsklinik Kiel
Arnold-Heller Strasse 7
D-2300 Kiel 1, FRG

H. Schillinger
Department of Obstetrics and Gynecology
Division of Clinical Endocrinology
University of Freiburg
D-7800 Freiburg-im-Breisgau, FRG

T. Schlotfeld
UKE Frauenklinik
Division of Endocrinology
Martinistrasse 52
2000 Hamburg 20, FRG

R. Scholler
Foundation de Recherche en
    Hormonologie
PB110
94268 Fresnes Cedex, France

John H. Seely
Abbott Laboratories
Abbott Park, IL 60064, USA

Tzuria Segal
Endocrinology Laboratory, Soroka
    Medical Center and
Division of Obstetrics and Gynecology
Clinical Biochemistry Unit, Faculty of
    Health Sciences
Ben Gurion University of the Negev
Beer-Sheba 84101, Israel

Yoav Sharoni
Endocrinology Laboratory, Soroka
    Medical Center and
Division of Obstetrics and Gynecology
Clinical Biochemistry Unit, Faculty of
    Health Sciences
Ben Gurion University of the Negev
Beer-Sheba 84101, Israel

R.W. Shaw
Academic Department of Obstetrics and
    Gynecology
Royal Free Hospital School of Medicine
London NW3, UK

R. Shiffl
Department of Internal Medicine
University of Heidelberg
Heidelberg, FRG

Karol Sikora
Department of Clinical Oncology
Hammersmith Hospital
DuCane Road
London W12 OHS, UK

M. Simmonds
Department of Medicine/Endocrinology
Milton S. Hershey Medical Center
Pennsylvania State University
PO Box 850, Hershey, PA 17033, USA

W.G. Sippell
Sophia Children's Hospital
160 Goodelweg
3038 GE Rotterdam, The Netherlands

Pierre C. Sizonenko
Department of Pediatrics and Genetics
Division of Biology of Growth and
    Reproduction
University of Geneva Medical School
1211 Geneva 4, Switzerland

P.H. Smith
A.Z. Middelheim
Antwerp 2020, Belgium

J. Smitz
Center for Reproductive Medicine
Medical Campus, Vrije Universiteit Brussel
Laarbeeklaan 101
1090 Brussels, Belgium

Y. Soffer
Department of Obstetrics and Gynecology
Assaf Harofe Medical Center
Zerefin, Israel

C. Staesson
Center for Reproductive Medicine
Medical Campus, Vrije Universiteit Brussel
Laarbeeklaan 101
1090 Brussels, Belgium

David Stephure
Department of Pediatrics
University of California San Francisco
San Francisco, CA 94943, USA

R. Strum
Klinik für Franenheilkunde und
    Geburtshilfe
Institut für Biochemische Endokrinologie
Medizinische Universiteit zu Lübeck
D-2400 Lübeck, FRG

Linda J. Swanson
Abbott Laboratories
Abbott Park, IL 60064, USA

R. Sylvester
A.Z. Middelheim
Antwerp 2020, Belgium

G.P. Taylor
Departments of Pediatrics and Pathology
University of British Columbia
BC's Children's Hospital
Vancouver, BC V6H 3V4, Canada

J.E. Toublanc
Foundation de Recherche en
    Hormonologie
PB110
94268 Fresnes Cedex, France

Ian Tummon
Section of Reproductive
    Endocrinology/Infertility
Department of Obstetrics and Gynecology
Rush Medical College
Chicago, IL 60612, USA

W.J. Tze
Department of Pediatrics and Pathology
University of British Columbia
BC's Children's Hospital
Vancouver, BC V6H 3V4, Canada

Wylie Vale
Salk Institute for Biological Studies
La Jolla, CA 92037, USA

A.N. van Geel
Department of Surgery
The Rotterdam Cancer Institute
Rotterdam, The Netherlands

A.C. Van Steirteghen
Center for Reproductive Medicine
Medical Campus, Vrije Universiteit Brussel
Laarbeeklaan 101
1090 Brussels, Belgium

L. Van Waesberghe
Center for Reproductive Medicine
Medical Campus, Vrije Universiteit Brussel
Laarbeeklaan 101
1090 Brussels, Belgium

Brian H. Vickery
Institute of Biological Sciences
Syntex Research
Palo Alto, CA 94304, USA

W. von Rechenberg
Hoechst AG
D-6230 Frankfurt 80, FRG

S. Waibel
Department of Obstetrics and Gynecology
Staedtische Kliniken
Grafenstrasse 9
D-6100 Darmstadt, FRG

H. Wand
Urologische Universitatsklinik Kiel
Arnold-Heller Strasse 7
D-2300 Kiel 1, FRG

Jonathan Waxman
Department of Clinical Oncology
Hammersmith Hospital
DuCane Road
London W12 OHS, UK

Gerhard F. Weinbauer
Max Planck Clinical Research Unit for
    Reproductive Medicine
Institute of Reproductive Medicine of the
    University
D-4400 Münster, FRG

Z. Weinraub
Department of Obstetrics and Gynecology
Assaf Hasofe Medical Center
Zerefin, Israel

J. Wettlaufer
Department of Medicine/Endocrinology
Milton S. Hershey Medical Center
Pennsylvania State University
PO Box 850, Hershey, PA 17033, USA

D. White-Hershey
Department of Medicine/Endocrinology
Milton S. Hershey Medical Center
Pennsylvania State University
PO Box 850, Hershey, PA 17033, USA

L. Wildt
Department of Gynecology and Obstetrics
University of Erlangen-Nürnberg
8520 Erlangen, FRG

G. Williams
Department of Urology
Hammersmith Hospital
DuCane Road
London W12 OHS, UK

A. Wisanto
Center for Reproductive Medicine
Medical Campus, Vrije Universiteit Brussel
Laarbeeklaan 101
1090 Brussels, Belgium

Arnon Wiznitzer
Endocrinology Laboratory, Soroka
    Medical Center and
Division of Obstetrics and Gynecology
Clinical Biochemistry Unit, Faculty of
    Health Sciences
Ben-Gurion University of the Negev
Beer-Sheba 84101, Israel

C. Wüster
Department of Internal Medicine
University of Heidelberg
Heidelberg, FRG

Attila Zalatnai
Veterans Administration Medical Center
1601 Perdido Street
New Orleans, LA 71046, USA

R. Ziegler
Department of Internal Medicine
University of Heidelberg
Heidelberg, FRG

1

THE USE OF LHRH ANALOGUES IN THE TREATMENT OF UTERINE FIBROIDS

D.L. HEALY
Medical Research Center, Monash Medical Center,
Prince Henry's Hospital Campus, Melbourne, Australia

INTRODUCTION

Uterine leiomyomata or fibroids are neoplasms of smooth muscle found in approximately 20% of women older than 30 years [1]. Fibroids are the most common tumour of the female genital organs and probably the most common tumour in women. Fibroids are commonly associated with infertility, menorrhagia and/or dysmenorrhea. Management of patients who have symptomatic uterine fibroids has traditionally been surgical: myomectomy for patients desirous of children or hysterectomy for women whose families are complete.

The availability of potent LHRH agonist compounds which initially enhance gonadotrophin release but then diminish gonadotrophin secretion upon continued administration has encouraged extensive investigation of LHRH agonists for use as novel drugs in the management of a spectrum of estrogen-dependent gynecological diseases [2]. LHRH analogues have been used to date in several small series of patients with uterine fibroids and this chapter reviews the current status of these agents in managing patients with this disease.

UTERINE FIBROIDS: THEIR GYNECOLOGICAL IMPACT

At a public health level, uterine fibroids constitute a major cost to gynecological care within health communities in the first world. This cost is the sum of medical attendances for symptomatic fibroids plus hospital costs for myomectomy and hysterectomy, the latter being the most common major operation performed in women. Table 1 indicates the rate of hysterectomy per 100,000 women in the United Kingdom, the United States of America and Australia: there is controversy about the reasons for the variable rates of hysterectomy in different countries and about the indications for such surgery [3]. Approximately 25%-50% of patients who undergo hysterectomy will sustain complications [4,5]. Most complications will be mild but haemorrhage, pelvic infection, sepsis and urinary tract injuries

Table 1. Hysterectomy rates per 100,000 women.

Country	Rate	Year	Reference
Scotland	213	1977	7
England and Wales	239	1977	7
U.S.A.	563	1980	8
Australia	613	1977	3

may occur. In the United States, the Committee on Gynecologic
Practice of the American College of Obstetricians and
Gynecologists has estimated hysterectomy-related deaths at over
600 per year from approximately 500,000 operations [6].
Moreover, significant psycho-social sequelae may follow
hysterectomy, including sexual dysfunction, loss of self-esteem
and alteration in a woman's perception of her own femininity.
    Uterine fibroids constitute the most common pathological
abnormality given as a reason for hysterectomy. In Scotland,
hysterectomy for fibroids was 21% of all hysterectomies in 1977
and 24% of all hysterectomies in England and Wales in that year
were performed for the same purpose [7]. In Australia,
fibroids were the reason given for hysterectomy in 40% of
patients [3].
    Public health costs associated with uterine fibroids are
significant. In the United States, it has been estimated that
over $1700 million dollars are spent for hysterectomy each year
[6]. In Australia, Federal Government Medicare benefits for
the calendar year 1986 indicated 21,000 items of hysterectomy
and myomectomy. Assuming that 40% of such hysterectomies were
for uterine fibroids [3], and adding the cost of in-patient
hospitalization, anaesthetic, operating theatre, nursing and
support services total costs of uterine fibroids to the
Australian community may be as much as $60 x 10^6 per year.

PATHOGENESIS OF UTERINE FIBROIDS

Uterine fibroids appear to be unicellular in origin, since each
of the cells comprising a leiomyoma contains the same
glucose-6- phosphate dehydrogenase enzyme [9]. The type of
enzyme may vary from one tumour to another within the same
uterus. Although it remains unclear why neoplastic
transformation occurs in some smooth muscle cells within the
uterus, several hormones may influence the rate of growth of
fibroid tumours.

Influence of Estradiol

Unopposed estrogen action is thought to be the strongest factor
in the pathogenesis of uterine fibroids. This belief is in
accord with the clinical findings that fibroids are most

commonly diagnosed in women aged between 30-40 years, that
fibroids tend to shrink after the menopause and that fibroids
can rapidly increase in size during pregnancy. In a long-term
follow up study, by the Oxford Family Planning Association, of
women using various methods of contraception, case-control
analysis of 535 women who had had a fibroid showed that the
risk of fibroids was inversely correlated with the number of
term pregnancies [10]. This suggested that low unopposed
estradiol levels, resulting from the several pregnancies and
also the subsequent puerperia, reduced the growth of nascent
fibroid tumours. The risk of developing uterine fibroids was
positively correlated with increasing duration of oral
contraceptive use, lower body weight and cigarette smoking.

In gynecological endocrine studies, several groups have
found that serum estradiol concentrations in women with uterine
fibroids were the same as those in control groups [12,13]. By
contrast, several reports have found higher concentrations of
estrogen receptors in fibroids than in normal myometrium of the
same uterus. Wilson and colleagues showed that estrogen and
progesterone receptor levels were increased in such tumours
when compared with adjacent myometrium but that the levels were
lower than those observed in endometrium from the same uterus
[14]. Soules and McCarty [13] also demonstrated more estrogen
and progesterone receptors in uterine fibroids, particularly
when measured in the follicular phase of the menstrual cycle
(estrogen receptor 33.6 ± 25.1 fmoles/mg protein in leiomyomas
cycle days 1-9 compared with 14.1 ± 2.6 normal myometrium).
More recently, Lumsden and associates reported estradiol
binding of 70 fmoles/mg protein in fibroids compared with a
median estradiol binding of 30 fmoles/mg protein in normal
uterine muscle [15].

Influence of Progesterone

Progesterone receptors have also been reported in uterine
fibroids and show cyclic changes throughout the menstrual cycle
similarly as found in endometrium [13]. Unlike estrogen
receptors, no clear increase in the relative amount of
progesterone binding sites in uterine fibroids has been
reported from such studies. Attempts to use progestogens in
the treatment of leiomyomas have not been generally
successful. Although Goldzieher and colleagues domonstrated
that large doses of the progestogen Medrogestone, 25 mg per day
given to patients for 3 weeks prior to hysterectomy, produced
degenerative changes in fibroids [16], other authors have been
unable to find evidence of involution of fibroids treated with
progesterone prior to hysterectomy [17]. More recently, the
estrogen and progesterone receptor antagonist, gestrinone, at
doses up to 5 mg twice weekly decreased uterine fibroid size
after treatment for 4-13 months [18]. These observations await
confirmation.

3

Local peptide growth factors

No consistent changes in circulating concentrations of growth hormones, human placental lactogen, insulin or other putative growth factors have been reported in patients with uterine fibroids. Nevertheless, the recent demonstration of local secretion of insulin-like growth factor 1 (IGF-1) and epidermal growth factor (EGF) within the ovary and the identification of IGF-1 receptors [19] suggests the possibility of additional local stimulators of fibroid growth (Table 2).

Table 2. Putative peptide growth factors for uterine fibroids.

Growth Factor	Competence Factor (Inducer)	Progression Factor (Promoter)
EGF (Epidermal)	X	
TGF-α (Transforming)	X	
Insulin	X	
IFG-I, IGF-II (Insulin-Like)	X	
PDGF (Platelet Derived)		X

LHRH AGONISTS FOR UTERINE FIBROIDS; PREDICTION OF RESPONSE

We have recently completed a controlled trial evaluating the LHRH agonist, buserelin, administered either intranasally or by subcutaneous infusion, in a group of 20 patients with symptomatic uterine fibroids. As shown in Table 3, addition of this data to published series of uterine fibroids treated with LHRH agonist indicates that 83% of fibroid tumours will become smaller with this treatment.

Precise definition of what constitutes shrinkage of uterine fibroids during LHRH agonist treatment has varied in these publications. We have defined significant shrinkage in the size of uterine fibroids in a patient as when the tumour volume decreases below 66% of the initial fibroid volume and when that shrinkage is confirmed by at least two consecutive observations.

We have treated 27 patients, aged 29-49 years, with symptomatic uterine fibroids manifested by menorrhagia, pressure symptoms, dysmenorrhea or otherwise unexplained infertility. Twenty subjects have completed 6 months of treatment. All had undergone curettage and had normal endometrial histology. Each patient had been individually assessed and independently diagnosed by other gynecologists to have uterine fibroids. All subjects were within 20% of ideal

4

Table 3. Published series of uterine fibroids treated with LHRH agonists.

Study	N	LHRH Agonist Used	Dose & Route	Response
Maheux et al '85 [20]	10	Buserelin	200 µg TDS S.C.	7
Coddington et al '86 [21]	6	[IMBZL-D-His^6 Pro^9-NHEt] LHRH	250 µg S.C.	6
Healy et al '86 [22]	5	Buserelin	200 µg S.C. infusion	5
Maheux et al '87 [23]	9	Buserelin	200 µg TDS S.C.; 400 µg TDS I.N.	8
Peal et al '87	10	[D-Trp^6] LHRH	500 µg S.C.; 100 µg S.C.	8
West et al '87	13	Zoladex	3-6 mg S.C. Implant	12
Healy et al '88	9	Buserelin	1200 µg I.N.	6
	11	Buserelin	200 µg S.C. Infusion	9
	73			61 (83%)

body weight and had taken no medication for at least two months. Individual patients' consent was obtained and the study was approved by the Research and Ethics Committees, Queen Victoria Medical Centre campus and Price Henry's Hospital campus, Monash Medical Centre. Tumour size in these patients ranged from 9 cm^3 in a woman with a cornual tumour and infertility to 953 cm^3 [3] in a thirty year old woman with menorrhagia and haemoglobin of 7.4 g % on referral. This latter tumour was equivalent in size to a 20 week pregnancy.

The LHRH agonist buserelin was supplied as buserelin acetate (1.50 mg/ml). It was administered as an intranasal spray by 12 x 100 µg insufflations per day, commencing on waking in the morning and spaced at regular intervals throughout the day until bedtime. For subcutaneous administration, buserelin was diluted in 0.9% sterile NaCl to provide an infusion of 200 µg per day or a bolus dose injected subcutaneously every 45 minutes [22].

Each patient commenced the study at approximately day 21 of a menstrual cycle. From day 1 of that cycle, and weekly thereafter, a 10 ml blood sample was obtained for determination of serum FSH, LH, E_2 and P. Commencement of buserelin treatment in the luteal phase was favoured following previous data indicating the time to menopausal serum E_2 concentrations (less than 50 pg/ml) was more rapid when LHRH agonist treatment was commenced then rather than in the follicular phase of the menstrual cycle [22,24,25].

Each patient underwent an initial gynecological examination to clinically estimate the size of the uterus and the uterine fibroids. In addition, fibroid volume was determined by ultrasound by an independent investigator. Scanning aspects of fibroid morphometry are detailed below. The dimensions of each fibroid in each patient were measured in three planes and the volume of all tumours was determined by the formula $4/3\pi R^3$, where R was the radius of the tumour for spherical fibroids or the product of length (d_1) by width (d_2) by depth (d_3) by 0.52 litre for tumours of other shapes. Ultrasound morphometry and gynecological examination were performed on at least one occasion before buserelin treatment and at 4- to 6-week intervals during treatment. Serum samples were stored at $-20°$ until assay for FSH, LH, E_2 and P using previously described methods [26,27]. Hormone radioimmunoassay quality control data for interassay variability, intraassay variability nd detection limit per ml were, respectively: FSH 4.9% at 5.6 IU/L; 4.1%; 0.2 IU/L: LH 5.4% at 8.0 IU/L; 3.5% 0.1 IU/L: E_2 9.1% at 500 pg/ml, 8.5% pg/ml: P 14.0% at 5.0 ng/ml, 9.8%; 0.2 ng/ml.

Table 4. Uterine fibroid volume during LHRH agonist treatment.

Weeks of Treatment	Fibroid Volume* (Mean $\pm$ SE)	Range
9.2 $\pm$ 0.5	72.0 $\pm$ 5.2 (n=20)	33.3–107.4
17.3 $\pm$ 0.5	60.8 $\pm$ 6.1 (n=15)	33.8–93.9
23.4 $\pm$ 0.3	49.6 $\pm$ 8.4 (n=13)	11.1–81.9

*Fibroid volume expressed as % of the initial tumour volume taken as 100%.

Table 4 shows fibroid volume as per ultrasound morphometry in our total group of patients on buserelin treatment, where the initial fibroid volume was expressed as 100% and subsequent fibroid volumes were expressed as a percentage of the patient's own initial tumour volume. In no patient was the fibroid tumour volume after 6 months of buserelin treatment greater than the initial fibroid volume. Eight of the 20 patients at the end of 6 months buserelin treatment had impalpable uterine fibroids on gynecological examination. Three of these patients had received intranasal buserelin treatment.

LHRH agonist treatment for uterine fibroids provides an in vivo opportunity to assess if fibroid growth in that

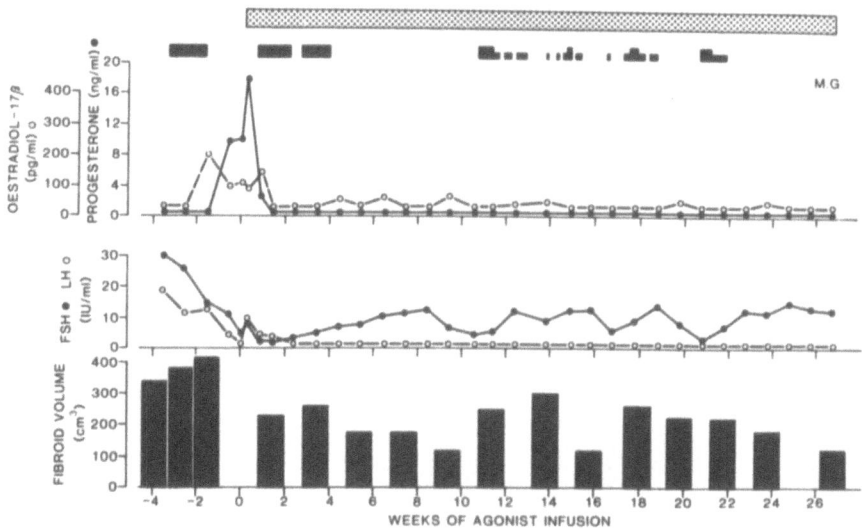

FIGURE 1   Endocrine and fibroid volume results in a patient
receiving intra-nasal buserelin for 6 months.

individual is responsive to circulating serum E_2
concentrations. Figures 1 and 2 depict 2 patients of similar
age with similar-sized fibroids. Intranasal buserelin
treatment administered to patient M.S. produced persistent
suppression of E_2 concentrations with no serum E_2 level
>50 pg/ml after the initial menstruation. Despite this, fibroid
volume did not decline below 80% of the initial tumour volume.
By contrast, patient M.G. demonstrated a decrease in fibroid
volume which was progressive and consistent down to a tumour
volume approximately 36% of the initial value. This occurred
despite E_2 concentrations which were in fact higher on
subcutaneous buserelin treatment than were observed in the
patient in Fig. 1. Note in both these climacteric patients the
relatively high serum FSH concentration. This compares with
the low FSH levels, together with LH values, observed in the
younger women receiving either intranasal or subcutaneous
buserelin treatment, as demonstrated by the 30-year-old patient
(Fig. 3).
     The consistent increase in the circulating FSH values
observed in older patients during this study confirms previous
observations in climacteric women. Although circulating E_2

7

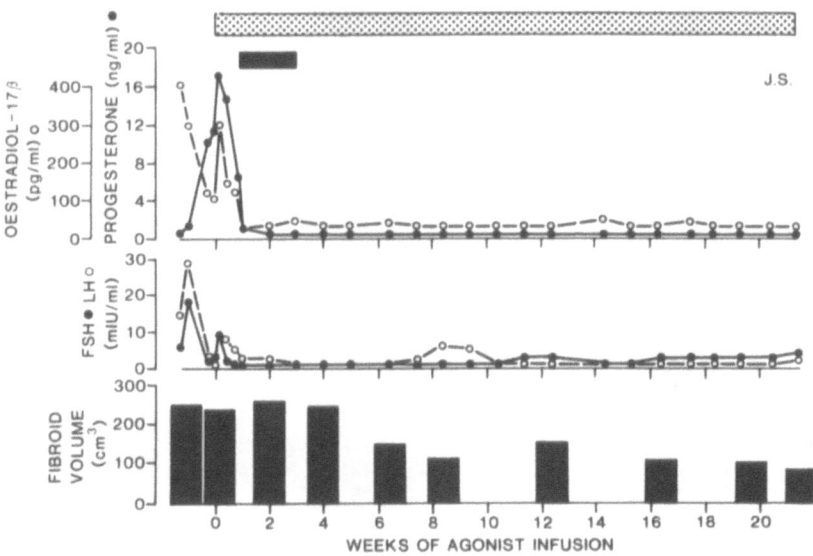

FIGURE 2   Endocrine and fibroid volume changes following
   intra-nasal buserelin treatment in a 30-year-old patient.

concentrations were statistically similar between young and
older women, the elevation in serum FSH levels was only
observed in the older patients.   Inhibin is an ovarian protein
which is known to suppress circulating FSH concentrations
[30].   Whether inhibin concentrations are lower in older
patients on buserelin treatment is not known at this time.
      These examples of persistent suppression of cyclic E_2
secretion from the ovary can be contrasted with other examples
of repetitive LHRH-agonist treatment.   Fig. 3 demonstrates
endocrine and fibroid responses in a patient receiving
subcutaneous buserelin treatment.   This patient showed a
cessation of cyclic gonadotrophin and steroid secretion for the
first 12 weeks of buserelin treatment.   Over weeks 13-15, a
small increase in both FSH and LH were observed and in week 18
a single serum E_2 concentration of 227 pg/ml was noted.   No
infusion pump malfunction was noted at this time in the subject
receiving subcutaneous treatment and the patient's compliance

8

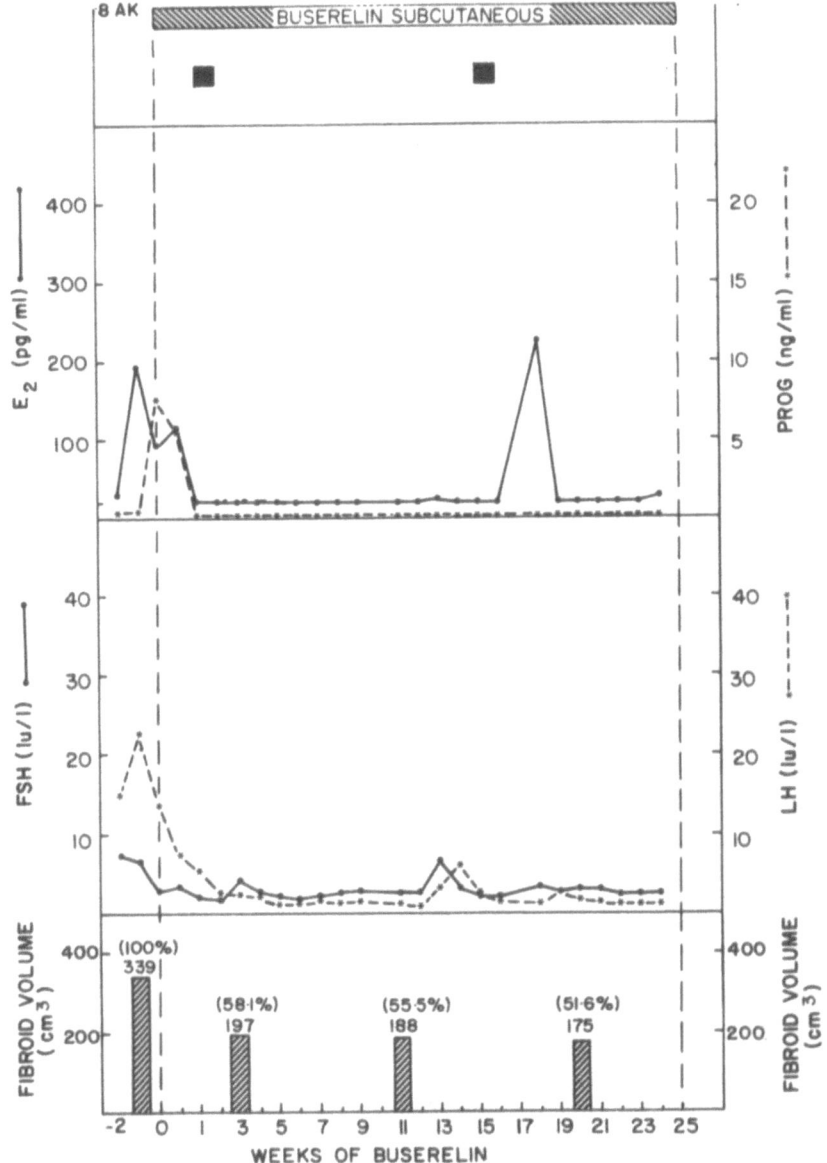

FIGURE 3 Endocrine and fibroid volume changes in a patient
receiving subcutaneous buserelin treatment.

9

was good. Treatment was maintained and serum E_2 values decreased and remained in the menopausal range until the end of treatment. There was no further elevation in serum FSH or LH concentrations.

Fig. 4 depicts results from another patient who showed episodes of significant serum E_2 secretion. The highest of these occurred between weeks 6-8 of buserelin treatment and they were not preceded by any significant increase in gonadotrophin values. No menstruation occurred at this time and E_2 values again decreased with no change in the intranasal buserelin dosage. Compliance was again judged to be satisfactory in this patient. Modest increases in LH were noted in week 14 in this subject, followed by a second E_2 peak at week 18 (464 pg/ml). This second E_2 elevation was followed by menstruation. These examples suggest escape from apparent pituitary desensitization and/or gonadotrophin-independent ovarian E_2 secretion. Escape from pituitary desensitization has previously been reported [22,28]. An alternative explanation for escape from the pituitary down-regulation that we observed in these patients would be that the E_2 secretion is gonadotrophin-independent. However, gonadotrophin-independent ovarian E_2 secretion has not previously been described in adult patients receiving LHRH-agonist treatment to our knowledge. Gonadotrophin-independent ovarian E_2 production has been previously reported in precocious puberty due to the McCune-Albright syndrome [29].

LHRH-agonists would be most valuable for the gynecological management of uterine fibroids if a series of clinical predictors of shrinkage and response were known. We have begun such a search for clinical predictors of response and Table 5 compares fibroid volume after repetitive intranasal or subcutaneous buserelin treatments. The fibroid volume in each patient group was averaged at 8, 16 and 24 weeks of administration. Tumour volume at each time decreased for each modality of treatment. There was no statistical difference between intranasal or subcutaneous therapy at any time. Intranasal buserelin treatment appeared equally as effective as subcutaneous administration of this drug. Of the 5 patients who failed to show a significant decrease in tumour volume 3 received intranasal and 2 received subcutaneous buserelin treatment.

Table 6 assesses uterine fibroid volume and buserelin treatment when analysed with respect to the initial tumour volume. Patients with a fibroid tumour volume <260 cm^3 on ultrasonography were compared with the other individuals. The larger tumours (>260 cm^3; approximately a fibroid 7 cm in diameter) appeared to show the greatest initial decrease in tumour size although at no time did the differences between large and small size tumours reach statistical significance.

Table 5. Effect of route of administration of LHRH-agonist
on fibroid tumour volume.

Weeks of Treatment	Fibroid Volume (Expressed as % of Initial Volume)	
	Intranasal	Subcutaneous
8	68.4 ± 10.1 (n=8)	74.9 ± 5.1 (n=10)
16	66.4 ± 9.3 (n=6)	56.1 ± 8.1 (n=7)
24	51.2 ± 14.4 (n=5)	48.3 ± 10.9 (n=6)

Mean ± SE.

Patients younger than 35 years with symptomatic uterine
fibroids will commonly present with infertility. The
availability of LHRH-agonists in this age group is potentially
of much gynecological value since the size of the tumour at
myomectomy has been regarded as an important prognostic factor
in subsequent fertility [31]. Table 7 compares the change in
fibroid volume in patients 35 years or younger with changes in
tumour volume in older women. At each assessment time (8, 16
or 24 weeks) the percentage decrease in fibroid volume was
greater in the younger women. This was especially evident
after 16 weeks of agonist treatment.

Table 6. LHRH-agonist and uterine fibroids: influence of
initial tumour size.

Weeks of Treatment	Fibroid Volume (Expressed as % of Initial Volume)	
	Initial Volume <260 cm^3	Initial Volume ≥260 cm^3
8	78.2 ± 7.6 (n=10)	64.3 ± 6.3 (n=8)
16	62.8 ± 8.1 (n=6)	59.2 ± 9.4 (n=7)
24	46.4 ± 11.0 (n=7)	55.2 ± 14.2 (n=4)

Mean ± SE.

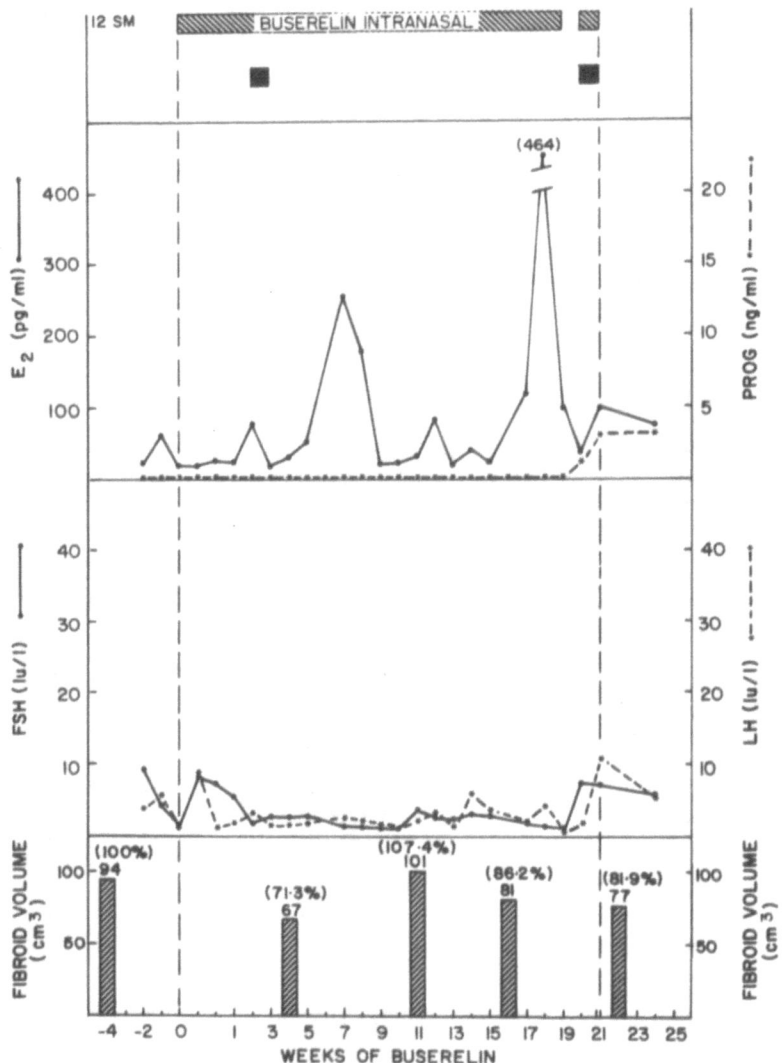

FIGURE 4   In this subject, serum E_2 levels were 265 pg/ml after 7 weeks of buserelin but this increase was not preceded by any obvious elevation in serum FSH or LH concentration. Similarly, no cyclic FSH and LH secretion was apparent before the serum E_2 level of 464 pg/ml on week 18 of treatment.

FIBROID ULTRASOUND MORPHOMETRY AND MYOMECTOMY

Ultrasound Morphometry

Uterine fibroids in our study were measured ultrasonically using an Aloka 280-SSD sector linear machine. Most measurements were made using a 3.5 mHz mechanical sector scanner. Measurements were made in 3 standard planes, the largest diameters being recorded from these supero-inferior, antero-posterior and transverse directions. To eliminate inter-observer bias amongst even experienced ultrasonographers [32], all ultrasound scans in our series were performed by a single observer. To minimise intra-observer bias, scans were performed without reference to any previous ultrasound results in the same patients.

As a further control, we undertook a pilot study using 4 patients with uterine fibroids who were about to undergo hysterectomy. Pre-operative measurements of the uterine fibroids were compared with actual measurements found in each hysterectomy specimen. This study showed that trans-vesical ultrasound measurements often overestimated the size of uterine fibroids because the area of compressed myometrium around the tumour was often included in the measurement. This error was greatest with large fibroids. Nevertheless, the overestimate was usually small (0.5-1.0 cm) and the study confirmed that trans-vesical abdominal ultrasound was a reliable method of measuring not only fibroid number and position but also fibroid size.

Table 7. LHRH-agonist and uterine fibroids: effect of patient age.

Weeks of Treatment	Fibroid Volume (Expressed as % of Initial Volume)	
	Age <35 Years	Age $\geq$35 Years
8	69.2 $\pm$ 4.8 (n=10)	75.5 $\pm$ 10.3 (n=8)
16	55.8 $\pm$ 6.5 (n=9)	72.1 $\pm$ 12.8 (n=4)
24	45.4 $\pm$ 14.2 (n=4)	52.1 $\pm$ 11.1 (n=7)

Mean $\pm$ SE.

This pre-hysterectomy study also highlighted some other difficulties for those aiming to undertake uterine fibroid morphometry. Firstly, a large fibroid may in fact be composed of a number of smaller tumours which, because of absorption of the ultrasound by the fibroids and the resultant decreased resolution, may not be seen as separate neoplasms. Secondly, and particularly with large fibroids, the adjacent normal uterus may not be seen separate from the tumour. In our experience, during treatment with LHRH-agonists, the fibroid becomes less ultrasonically visible as the endometrium becomes less prominent. After cessation of treatment and the establishment of normal menstrual cycles, these changes reverse. Thirdly, although some fibroids appear initially irregular in outline, they are in fact spherical with the irregular appearance being due to the presence of a number of smaller tumours. Finally, although some fibroids in our series showed calcific and other degenerative changes before LHRH-agonist commenced, the development of degenerative changes within the interstices of a fibroid have not usually been apparent from our studies. This is despite significant hyaline or cystic degeneration within the tumour when examined after removal at myomectomy or hysterectomy. On the other hand, development of calcification within a fibroid can be reliably recognized.

Myomectomy

Traditional surgical technique for uterine myomectomy includes pressure on the uterine vessels before myomectomy [1,31,33]. This usually requires dissection of the bladder from the lower segment of the uterus and placement of a myomectomy clamp or tourniquet. Both these procedures risk damage to the pelvic peritoneum and/or uterine tube with subsequent adhesion formation, compromising future fertility.

We have undertaken myomectomy in an infertile patient at the end of 6 months of buserelin treatment. Fibroid volume had decreased to 56.6% of initial volume in this subject and no ultrasonic evidence of degeneration or calcification within the tumour was noted. At laparotomy, no grossly dilated vessels over the surface of the fibroid were seen. A midline incision over the least vascular part of the uterus was able to be performed using blended cutting/coagulation diathermy without the need for a myomectomy clamp or other tourniquet upon the uterine or ovarian blood vessels. Morever, dissection of the serosa from the fibroid could also be performed with satisfactory hemostasis. Although this was a large tumour requiring resection almost to the endometrium the fibroid could be removed and the dead space obliterated in this hypo-estrogenic uterus without the usual blood loss which attends significant myomectomy. Histopathology of this tumour showed extensive hyaline degeneration in the centre of the neoplasm which was well demarcated and possibly related to the effect of hypo-estrogenism and buserelin therapy. Conception occurred 4 weeks after myomectomy and an intra-uterine pregnancy was confirmed.

Pre-operative use of LHRH-agonists prior to myomectomy may allow fibroid myomectomy to be performed with improved hemostasis and with reduced morbidity due to less risk of abrasive damage to the pelvic peritoneum or uterine tubes from uterine clamps or tourniquets. Combined medical-surgical approaches to the management of uterine fibroids in the young or infertile patient now appears feasible.

COMPLIANCE AND SIDE EFFECTS

Only one of 27 patients in our 6-month study which required weekly attendance for medical care, has terminated buserelin treatment due to poor compliance. That 26 of 27 patients were compliant with such a strenuous protocol was surprising. After 6 months treatment, patients were asked to assess the treatment they received, either intranasal insufflation or subcutaneous infusion, as a possible treatment for uterine fibroids and also to assess how they might rate a future LHRH-agonist implant treatment, requiring only a single injection every 8 weeks. On a scale of 10 in this pilot study in which 10 represented completely suitable, the mean score for either intranasal or subcutaneous infusion was 8 while all patients believed an LHRH-agonist implant system would be completely suitable from their viewpoint in an attempt to avoid laparotomy.

All patients receiving either intranasal or subcutaneous buserelin treatment for uterine fibroids developed hot flushes. Typically, these began 4 weeks after the commencement of LHRH- agonist treatment (range 2-7 weeks) and reached peak frequency at 6 weeks of therapy. The frequency of hot flushes then decreased in most patients although 3 of 18 subjects required hypnotics to induce sleep because of continuing troublesome hot flushes. No patient requested cessation of buserelin treatment because of incapacitating hot flushes.

No patient continued to suffer menorrhagia while on LHRH-agonist treatment. Twelve of 20 subjects were amenorrheic following the first steroid withdrawal menstruation which began approximately 7 days after commencing buserelin treatment. In the remaining 8 individuals, light vaginal bleeding or spotting occurred during treatment.

Four patients described persistent joint pains during buserelin treatment. In each case, patients described symptoms in the proximal and distal interphalangeal joints of the hands which were typically worse in the dominant hand. One subject was reviewed by a rheumatologist who diagnosed flexor tenosynovitis aggravated by employment and prescribed a non-steroidal anti-inflammatory drug which produced improvement in joint pain. Buserelin treatment continued throughout this time. The three other patients did not require specific treatment.

One subject was withdrawn from buserelin treatment due to persistent nasal congestion and rhinorrhoea. This patient received intranasal buserelin and was well for the first 16 weeks of treatment. At that time, a persistently stuffy nose

15

and nasal discharge occurred. The patient herself ceased intranasal buserelin spray during week 19 of the trial with an improvement in her symptoms. She then recommenced the spray at the end of that week with a recurrence of the same symptoms. Intranasal buserelin was ceased in this subject after 21 weeks of treatment. The patient remained well after that time and all nasal symptoms resolved. However, since stopping LHRH-agonist treatment, this individual has had further heavy menorrhagia.

Radial cortical bone thickness was measured by single photon densitometry in 10 subjects before and after 6 months of buserelin treatment for uterine fibroids. Pre-buserelin bone density was 459 $\pm$ 21 mg/ml (mean $\pm$ SE; range 392-521) while radial cortical bone thickness after 6 months' buserelin treatment was 431 $\pm$ 18 (385-487). In this pilot study, physical activity and oral calcium intake were not controlled. Such factors may be important in relatively young patients receiving chronic LHRH-agonist treatment where potentially more sensitive indices of bone mineral loss, such as CT scans of the lumbar vertebrae and estimates of total body calcium by neutron activation have yielded conflicting results concerning the bone loss observed with LHRH-agonist therapy [34,35,36]. This issue requires further investigation as does the assessment of lipid and lipoprotein changes in patients receiving chronic LHRH-agonist treatment.

FUTURE DIRECTIONS

LHRH-agonists provide for the first time a medical treatment for uterine fibroids. LHRH-agonists significantly shrink these tumours in the majority of patients and causes them to clinically disappear in some. The potential impact of such treatment upon current gynecological care of patients with uterine fibroids may be significant. Such impact may be at various levels, especially with the pending availability of suitable implant systems of LHRH-agonists for chronic gynecological disease such as fibroids or endometriosis.

Pre-operative use of LHRH-agonists prior to myomectomy for uterine fibroids seems a treatment of choice. Patients less than 35 years appear particularly suitable because shrinkage of fibroids is more consistent in this age group. Such patients are also more likely to complain of infertility and in these circumstances reduction of estrogen-dependent uterine blood flow, as well as the reduction in tumour size, are both important surgical advantages. LHRH-analogues may also allow a less invasive surgical operation.

Use of LHRH-analogues as definitive treatment for uterine fibroids can also now be explored. Our results, and those of other investigators, suggest that approximately one third of patients receiving LHRH-agonists for this condition will have their tumours clinically disappear after 6 months therapy.

Although tumours do regrow in the majority of patients, following cessation of therapy, it is not yet clear whether symptoms also return at a similar rate. This is of great clinical importance and LHRH-agonist treatment may alleviate pressure symptoms and menorrhagia in a relatively large number of middle-aged or climacteric patients. Moreover, the use of adjunctive medical treatment either with progestogens or estrogen receptor antagonists, such as tamoxifen, in patients with a significant decrease in tumour size after a course of LHRH-agonist treatment can now be studied.

LHRH-agonist availability has also advanced understanding of the pathogenesis of this most common neoplasm in women. Chronic use of intranasal or subcutaneous LHRH-agonists, or the pending widespread availability of biodegradable lactide-glycolide copolymers which can be injected as a single subcutaneous injection every 4 or 8 weeks [37], provides a hypo-estrogenic environment that distinguishes fibroids which are estrogen- dependent from those which are not. Furthermore, such medicines have been used in related tumours, such as benign metastasizing leiomyoma [38]. Potential medical therapy not only for fibroids and other benign tumours, but also for leiomyosarcomas may now be possible, offering new options for gynecological management.

ACKNOWLEDGEMENTS

The assistance of Prof. Carl Wood, Prof. John Leeton, Mr. Arthur Day, Dr. John Campbell, Dr. Gab Kovacs, Dr. Elizabeth Farrell and Dr. Kate Duncan at the Monash Medical Centre who provided patients for this study is gratefully acknowledged. Joan Williams and Jenny Judd provided excellent typing skills.

REFERENCES

1.   Dewhurst, CJ (ed.) (1981).   Integrated Obstetrics and Gynecology for Postgraduates. (Blackwell; London)
2.   McLachlan, RI, Healy, DL and Burger, HG (1986). Clinical aspects of LHRH analogues in gynecology: a review. Brit J Obstet Gynecol, 93, 431
3.   Opit, LJ and Gadiel, (1982). Hysterectomy in NSW. Office of Health Care Finance, Sydney
4.   Thompson, JD and Barch, HW (1981). Indications for hysterectomy. Clin Obstet Gynecol, 24, 1245
5.   Dicker, RC, Greenspan, JR, Strauss, LT, Cowart, MR, Scally, MJ, Peterson, HB, DeStefano, F, Rubin, GL and Ory, HW (1982). Complications of abdominal and vaginal hysterectomy among women of reproductive age in the United States. Am J Obstet Gynecol, 144, 841
6.   Easterday, CL, Grimes, DA and Riggs, JA (1983). Hysterectomy in the United States. Obstet Gynecol, 62, 203

7.   Cole, SK (1984). The Information Services Division of
the Scottish Health Service (personal communication)
8.   National Center for Health Statistics (1982). Vital and
Health Statistics, 1982, Series 13, Number 64
9.   Townsend, DE, Sparkes, RS, Baluda, MC and McClelland, G
(1970). Unicellular histogenesis of uterine leiomyomas as
determined by electrophoresis of glucose-6-phosphate
dehydrogenase. Am J Obstet Gynecol, 107, 1168
10.   Ross, RK, Pike, NC, Vessey, NP, Bull, D, Yates, D and
Casagrande, JT (1986). Risk factors for uterine fibroids:
reduced risk associated with oral contraceptives. Brit Med J,
293, 359
11.   Henderson, BE, Casagrande, JT and Pike, NC (1983). The
epidemiology of endometrial cancer in young women. Brit J
Cancer, 47, 749
12.   Spellacy, WN, Lemaire, WJ, Buhl, WC, Birk, SA and
Bradley, BA (1972). Plasma growth hormone and estradiol levels
in women with uterine myomas. Obstet Gynecol, 40, 829
13.   Soules, MR and McCarty, KS (1982). Leiomyomas: steroid
receptor content. Am J Obstet Gynecol, 143, 6
14.   Wilson, BA, Wang, F and Rees, ED (1980). Estradiol and
progesterone binding in uterine leiomyomata and in normal
uterine tissues. Obstet Gynecol, 55, 20
15.   Lumsden, MA, West, CP, Hawkins, TA, Rumgay, L and Baird,
DT (1987). The binding of steroids to human myometrium and
leiomyomata. Program of the Society for the Study of
Fertility, July 6-9, Abstract 30
16.   Goldzieher, JW, Maqueo, M, Ricaud, L, Aguilar, AJ and
Canale, SE (1966). Induction of degenerative changes in
uterine myomas by high dose progestin therapy. Am J Obstet
Gynecol, 96, 1078
17.   Segaloff, A, Weed, JC, Sternberg, WH and Parson, W
(1949). The progesterone therapy of human uterine leiomyomas.
J Clin Endocrinol Metab, 9, 1273
18.   Coutinho, EM, Baulanger, GA and Goncalvas, MT (1986).
Regression of uterine leiomyomas after treatment with
gestrinone, and antiestrogen, antiprogesterone. Am J Obstet
Gynecol, 155, 761
19.   Adashi, EY, Resnick, CE, D'Ercole, AJ, Szerboda, ME and
Van Wyke, JJ (1985). Insulin-like growth factors as
intraovarian regulators of granulosa cell growth and function.
Endocr Rev, 6, 400
20.   Maheux, R, Guilloteau, C, Lemay, A, Bastide, A and
Fazekas, ATA (1985). Luteinizing hormone-releasing hormone
agonist and uterine leiomyoma: a pilot study. Am J Obstet
Gynecol, 152, 1034
21.   Coddington, CC, Collins, RL, Shawker, TH, Anderson, R,
Loriaux, DL and Winkel, CA (1986). Long-acting gonadotrophin
hormone-releasing hormone analogues used to treat uteri.
Fertil Steril, 45, 624
22.   Healy, DL, Lawson, FR, Abbott, M and Baird, DT (1986).
Toward removing uterine fibroids without surgery: subcutaneous

infusion of a luteinizing hormone-releasing hormone agonist
commencing in the luteal phase. J Clin Endocrinol Metab, <u>63</u>,
619

23.   Maheux, R, Lemay, A and Merat, P (1987). The use of
intranasal luteinizing hormone-releasing hormone agonist in
uterine leiomyomas. Fertil Steril, <u>47</u>, 229

24.   Fraser, HM and Sandow, J (1985). Suppression of
follicular maturation by infusion of a luteinizing
hormone-releasing hormone agonist starting during the late
luteal phase in the stumped-tailed Macaque monkey. J Clin
Endocrinol Metab, <u>60</u>, 579

25.   McLachlan, V, Besanko, M, Wade, H, O'Shea, F, Frounson,
AO, and Healy, DL (1988). LHRH agonist treatment in previously
resistant patients undergoing in vitro fertilization. IVF (in
press) 1987. Jones, HW (ed.), New York Academy of Science (in
press)

26.   Okamoto, S, Healy, DL, Howlett, DT, Rogers, PAW, Leeton,
JF, Trounson, AO and Wood, EC (1986). An analysis of plasma
estradiol concentrations during clomiphene citrate - human
menopausal gonadotrophin stimulation in an in vitro
fertilization - embryo transfer programme. J Clin Endocrinol
Metab, <u>63</u>, 736

27.   Sufi, SBA, Donaldson, A and Jeffcoate, SL (eds.) (1985).
Programme for the provision of matched assay reagents for the
radioimmunoassay for hormones in reproductive physiology.
(Method Manual, Ninth Edition; WHO, Geneva)

28.   Kerl, ED, Williams, G, Hare, H and Bloom, SR (1984).
Failure of long-term luteinizing releasing hormone treatment
for prostatic cancer to suppress serum luteinizing hormone and
testosterone. Brit Med J, <u>289</u>, 468

29.   Comite, F, Shawker, TH, Pescovitz, OH, Loriaux, DL and
Cutler, GB (1984). Cyclical ovarian function resistant to
treatment with an analogue of luteinizing hormone releasing
hormone in McCune-Albright syndrome. New Engl J Med, <u>311</u>, 1032

30.   McLachlan, RI, Robertson, DM, Healy, DL, de Kretser, DM
and Burger, HG (1986). Plasma inhibin levels during
gonadotrophin- induced ovarian hyperstimulation for IVF. A new
index of follicular function? Lancet, <u>i</u>, 1233

31.   Buttram, VC and Reiter, RC (1981). Uterine leiomyomata:
etiology, symptomatology and management. Fertil Steril, <u>36</u>, 433

32.   Eissa, ML, Hudson, K, Docker, MF, Sawers, RS and Newton,
JR (1985). Ultrasound follicle diameter measurement: an
assessment of interobserver and intraobserver variation.
Fertil Steril, <u>44</u>, 751

33.   Howkins, J and Stallworthy, J (1974). Bonney's
Gynecological Surgery, 8th Edition, p. 410 (Bailliere Tindall;
London)

34.   Cedars, M, Steingold, K, Lu, J, Randel, ED, Meldrum, D
and Judd, H (1987). Treatment of endometriosis with a
long-acting GnRH agonist (GnRH-A) and medroxyprogesterone
acetate (MPA). Program of Society of Gynecologic Investigation
34th Annual Meeting, March 18-21, 1987, Abstract 289

35.   Lewis, V, Ramos, J and Darwood, Y (1987). Changes in bone mineral content in endometriosis patients treated with GnRH agonist. Program of Society of Gynecologic Investigation 34th Annual Meeting, March 18-21, 1987, Abstract 297

36.   Kenigsberg, D, Hull, M, Yasumara, S, Cohn, and Ellis, K (1987). Total body calcium (TBC) by neutron activation (NA) and osteocalcin (OC) in GnRH agonist (GnRHa) treated women with endometriosis. Program of Society of Gynecologic Investigation 34th Annual Meeting, March 18-21, 1987, Abstract 195

37.   West, CP, Lumsden, MA, Lawson, S, Williamson, J and Baird, DT (1987). Shrinkage of uterine fibroids during therapy with goserelin (Zoladex): a luteinizing hormone-releasing hormone agonist administered as a monthly subcutaneous depot. Fertil Steril, 48, 45

38.   Hague, WM, Abdul Wahid, NA, Jacobs, HS and Kraft, I (1986). Use of LHRH analogue to obtain reversible castration in a patient with benign metastisizing leiomyoma. Brit J Obstet Gynecol, 93, 455

2

TREATMENT OF UTERINE FIBROIDS WITH INTRA-NASAL BUSERELIN

R. ERNY, E. MILLIET and **L. BOUBLI**
Gynecologie – Obstetrique, Hôpital Michel Levy, Annexe Conception,
84a, rue de Lodi, 13281 Marseille Cedex 6, France

INTRODUCTION

The repeated subcutaneous or intranasal administration of GnRH
analogs leads to a paradoxical inhibition of the pituitary-ovarian
axis. This desensitization is rapidly reversible after
treatment. Such a temporary castration can offer a medical
treatment of uterine fibroids that could be comparable to the
important decrease in size of leiomyoma after menopause.

After having observed a favorable response of an uterine
fibroid under GnRH agonist therapy, Maheaux et al [1] investigated
LHRH agonists in this indication. They noted a marked decrease in
size of the leiomyomas and a gain in fertility of these infertile
women. However, this good efficacy is transient; leiomyomas
rapidly recover their initial size after treatment.

Other authors, have also studied LHRH agonists in this
indication [2-5]. The aim of the present study was to further
assess the place of these analogs in the treatment of uterine
fibroids.

MATERIAL AND METHODS

Fifteen women, aged 18 to 45 , presenting with uterine fibroids
have been included in this study. All had been informed and had
given their oral consent. The possibility of avoiding surgery or
desire of pregnancy strongly motivated them.

Only one patient dropped out of the study, at month 2,
because of personal reasons, not for side-effect.

The results are preliminary. They only concern 11 out of 15
patients who have completed the 6 month therapy. Five of them
have been followed during a 6 month period. Further study will be
required to assess relapse rate.

All patients underwent a complete clinical examination
before treatment, including cervical smear, and pelvic ultrasonography. The diagnosis was confirmed and the exact sizes of the
uterine fibroids measured. Biological investigations included

liver enzyme and hormonal assessments (E_2, FSH, LH and PRL).
Buserelin was given intranasally at the dose of 300µg, three times a day for 6 months.
Patients were checked regularly, at 3 weeks and 2, 4, and 6 months of treatment. A clinical, biological and hormonal examination was carried out at each visit. The size of the fibroid was also measured. Patients were questioned about compliance and side effects at month 6.

RESULTS

A. Fibroid size

The fibroid volumes decreased during LHRH analog treatment. The mean diameter decreased from 42 ±3mm before treatment, to 37 ± 3mm at month 2 and 33 ± 3 at month 6 (Fig. 1).

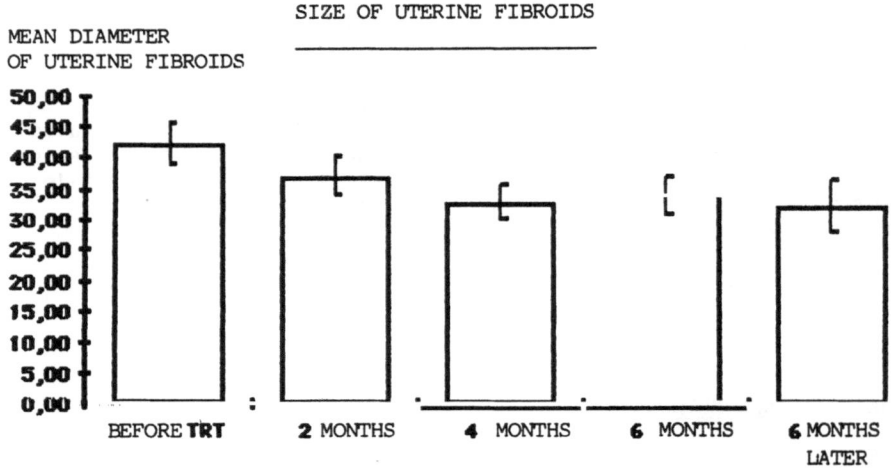

FIGURE 1   Change in size of uterine fibroids during and after treatment with buserelin.

The decrease appears as soon as the second month of treatment, is maximal at month 4 and is stable thereafter.
In one patient, the fibroid became necrotic and was easily extracted after cervical ripening. After surgery the uterus had a totally normal aspect.

B. Bleeding

We noted the disappearance of menstruation in the first month of treatment. However some patients reported small amounts of blood loss during therapy. Their mean duration was of 3 days: 3.7 during the first month, 3.2 during the second, 5.3 during the third and fourth and 1.9 during the last two.
    For each patient, the treatment was begun on the first day of the cycle; blood loss often occured 10 to 15 days later. Except for the necrosis, blood loss during the study was related to a few cases of bad compliance. After treatment, cycles reappeared 21 to 40 days later, with a mean of 30 days.

C. Hormonal investigations

After flare-up, FSH, LH and E_2 were at follicular phase levels (Figs. 2 and 3).

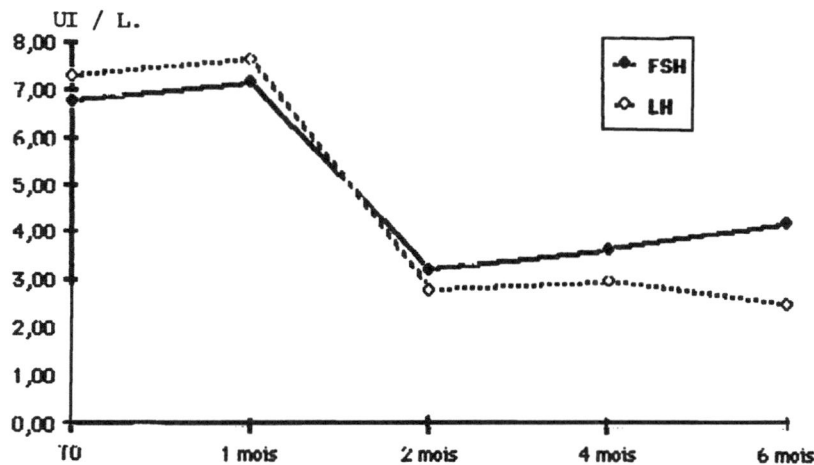

FIGURE 2   Values for LH and FSH during 6 months of treatment with buserelin.

    No change was noted for the other biological parameters.

D. Safety

Compliance has been very strong because of the patients'

motivation. Hot flushes occurred within the first month. They
were reported by 9 patients out of 11, severe in 6. They
disappear after drug withdrawal. Headaches were reported by 9
patients; they were not severe except in 2 cases. Vaginal
dryness, mood changes, dizziness and trouble with sleeping were
mentioned in very few cases. Patients were happy not to put on
weight. Only hot flushes have bothered the patients. Their
opinion on the treatment was favorable.

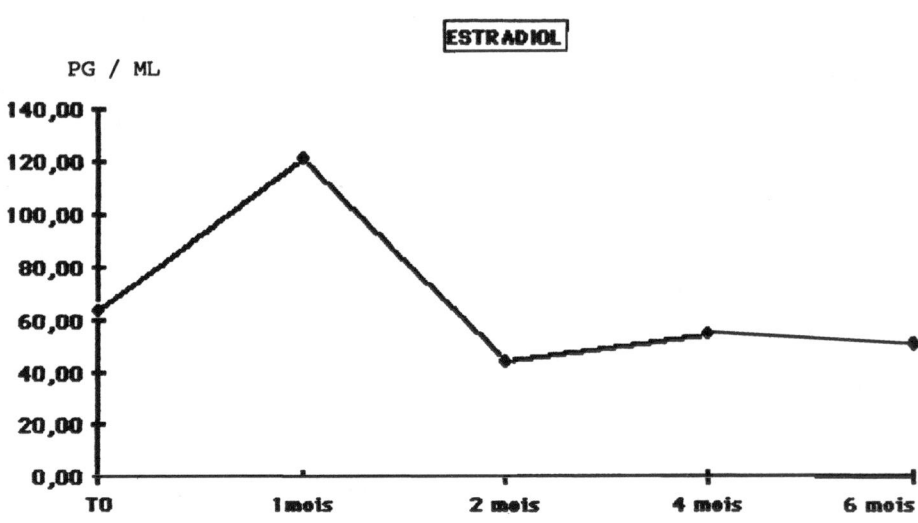

FIGURE 3   Values for serum estradiol during 6 months treatment
        with buserelin.

DISCUSSION

The benefit from intranasal buserelin appears at the second month
and is maximal at month 4. Further fibroid volume decrease does
not continue during the last 2 months. Four months can therefore
be considered to be the optimal time of treatment.

    The mean decrease is 22%, the maximum being 40%. The
interindividual variation is quite important. The reduction in
fibroid volume in this study is slightly less than that reported
by other authors [3, 5-7]. Maheux et al had noted a mean decrease
of 71% with intranasal buserelin started after 3 weeks of

subcutaneous administration [1]. The effects described by Rolland et al were also marked (26 to 71%) [4]. Some authors [8] showed that the decrease in volume was related to the oestradiol level: therefore, drugs administered subcutaneously might have a greater efficacy than when inhaled 3 times a day, due to better compliance.

Three questions remain: 1) Should all fibroids be treated? This is not justified when there is no malignant evolution. Two thirds of fibroids never need treatment. Treatment benefit is not often maintained long enough. 2) Systematic medical treatment before surgery? LHRH agonist are safe. Cessation of blood loss corrects anemia, prevents transfusion and makes post operative follow-up easier. Reduction of fibroid masses allows vaginal surgery which can take place after 3 or 4 month treatment. 3) Is the treatment by LHRH agonist relevant? Yes, in case of infertility. After a literature review, Buttram has estimated relapse after surgery to be about 15% [9]. Ramdomized studies are necessary, however, it is not relevant to treat small asymtomatic fibroids. Pre and post surgery treatment is certainly relevant for young or infertile women.
 For older patients, with no desire for pregnancy, treatment with LHRH agonists can allow vaginal surgery; necrobiosis can then prevent hysterectomy. LHRH agonists are very useful when a contra-indication prevents surgery and when, at the age of pre-menopause, a hormonal treatment is not suitable.

REFERENCES

1.   Maheux, R, Guilloteau, C, Lemay, A, Bastide, A, and Fezekas, ATA (1984). Regression of leimyomata uteri following hypoestrogenism induced by repetitive LHRH agonist treatment: preliminary report. Fertil Steril, 42, 644
2.   Coddington, CC, Collins, RL, Shawken, TH, Anderson, R, Loriaux, DL and Winkel, CA (1986). Long acting gonadotropin hormone releasing hormone analog used to treat uteri. Fertil Steril, 45, 624
3.   Lumsden, MA, West, C and Baird, DT (1987). Goserelin therapy before surgery for uterine fibroids. Lancet, 1, 8523
4.   Rolland, R, Franssen, AM, Willemsen, WN and Corbey, RS (1986). Uterine leiomyoma and LHRH agonist treatment. A preliminary report. In "Gonadotropin down regulation in gynecological practice". p.313. (New York: Alan R. Liss)
5.   Van Leusden, HAIM (1986). Rapid reduction of uterine myomas after short term treatment with micro encapsulated D-Trp^{6}LHRH. Lancet, 2, 8517
6.   Maheux, R and Lemay, A (1986). Uterine leiomyoma: treatment with LHRH agonist gonadotropin down regulation in gynecological practice. p.247 (New York: Alan R Liss)
7.   Perl, V, Marquez, J, Schally, AV, Comaru-Schally, AM, Leal, G, Zacharias, S and Gomes-Lira, C (1987). Treatment of leimyomata uteri with DTRP 6 luteinizing hormone releasing hormone. Fertil Steril, 48, 3, 383

8.   Friedman, AJ, Barbieri, RL, Benacerraf, BR and Schiff, I
(1987). Treatment of leiomyomata with intra nasal or subcutaneous
leuprolide, a gonadotropin releasing hormone agonist. Fertil
Steril, 48, 560
9.   Buttram, VC (1986). Uterine Leimomyomata Oetiology,
symptomatology and management. "Gonadotropin down Regulation in
Gynecological Practice". p.275 (New York: Alan R Liss)

3

ADVANCES IN THE TREATMENT OF LEIOMYOMATA UTERI WITH LEUPROLIDE

Andrew J. FRIEDMAN
Brigham and Women's Hospital, Fertility and Endocrine Unit,
75 Francis Street, Boston, Massachusetts 02115, USA

INTRODUCTION

Uterine leiomyomata or fibroids are the most common solid pelvic tumors found in women of reproductive age. Approximately 20-25% of women develop leiomyomata and 20-50% of these women will experience symptoms due to these tumors [1-5]. The most common symptoms include menorrhagia, pelvic pressure (i.e., urinary frequency, constipation), pelvic pain, and the appreciation of a pelvic mass. Until recently, leiomyomata were managed by primary surgical therapy: hysterectomy or myomectomy. Hysterectomy is the most common surgical treatment for leiomyomata and approximately 200,000 women undergo this procedure each year for fibroids in the United States alone [6]. Myomectomy can also be performed for leiomyomata in women requiring treatment who wish to maintain childbearing potential.

The discovery of gonadotropin releasing-hormone agonists (GnRH-a) and their ability to induce a pseudomenopausal, hypoestrogenic state has led to widespread clinical trials in the treatment of hormonally-dependent disease states in women. Because an estrogenic milieu appears necessary for the development and growth of leiomyomata [7,8], GnRH-a have been successfully employed in several studies to induce regression of uterine and leiomyomata volume [9-14]. The goals of GnRH-a therapy in the treatment of uterine fibroids have been to reduce the need for primary surgical therapy and to serve as a surgical adjunct, potentially reducing operative risk, in those patients undergoing hysterectomy or myomectomy.

I will summarize two recent trials [9,10] utilizing leuprolide acetate (TAP Pharmaceuticals, North Chicago, IL) in the treatment of leiomyomata uteri. In the first study, the efficacy of two delivery systems (intranasal spray versus subcutaneous injections) was compared. In the second study, the efficacy of subcutaneous leuprolide acetate with or without medroxyprogesterone acetate (MPA) was compared.

SUBCUTANEOUS VERSUS INTRANASAL LEUPROLIDE ACETATE IN THE TREATMENT OF LEIOMYOMATA

In a study [9] comparing two delivery systems of leuprolide acetate in the treatment of leiomyomata uteri, 14 premenopausal women were randomized to receive either subcutaneous (SC) or intranasal (IN) leuprolide. Seven patients received daily self-administered SC leuprolide acetate 0.5 mg for 24 weeks; seven other patients received leuprolide acetate 0.8 mg twice daily by IN spray for 23 weeks following a "loading dose" of SC leuprolide acetate 0.5 mg daily for 1 week. Initiation of therapy was within the first 3 days of menses in both groups.

All 7 women in the SC group completed the 24 week treatment protocol whereas only 3 of 7 women in the IN group finished. The poor completion rate in the IN group was due to the persistence of presenting symptoms (Table 1). All patients in the SC group were

Table I. Symptoms pretreatment and at 24 weeks of therapy in women with leiomyomata treated with subcutaneous (SC) or intranasal (IN) leuprolide acetate

	SC (n=7)			IN (n=7)		
	Pre-treatment	Week 24	Percent Resolution	Pre-treatment	Week 24	Percent Resolution
Menorrhagia	3	0	100%	3	2	33%
Pelvic pressure	4	0	100%	3	3	0%
Pelvic pain	-	-	-	1	1	0%

markedly hypoestrogenic, estradiol (E_2)<30 pg/ml, by 4 weeks of therapy and had resolution of their presenting symptoms by 12 weeks. In addition, all 7 SC patients achieved amenorrhea by 4 weeks of therapy. Only 3 of 7 IN patients developed amenorrhea with the remaining 4 patients experiencing vaginal bleeding ranging from intermittent spotting to heavy flow. Serum E_2 levels in the IN group ranged from 50-164 pg/ml. The inability of the IN-delivered leuprolide to adequately suppress E_2 levels was attributed to poor absorption of the drug through the nasal mucosa [15].

In the SC group, mean uterine volume decreased by 45% at 12 weeks of therapy (Table 2). By 24 weeks, a mean reduction of 53% in uterine volume was noted. The difference in uterine volumes at 12 and 24 weeks was not statistically significant. In the IN group, no statistical change in uterine volume occurred during the 24 week treatment period. When the data from both groups were pooled at 12 weeks of therapy, the percent reduction in uterine volume was negatively correlated with serum E_2 levels ($r=-0.55$, $P<0.05$). Bone density, measured by single photon absorptiometry

Table 2. Percent change in uterine volume during treatment with subcutaneous leuprolide and after 4 months of follow-up

	Uterine Volume (cm^3) (n=7)	Percent of Pretreatment Uterine Volume
Pretreatment	368 ± 60[a]	100.0
12 weeks therapy	202 ± 61[b]	55.0
24 weeks therapy	172 ± 49[b]	46.8
4 months post-therapy	296 ± 104	80.5

[a]Mean ± standard error
[b]$p < 0.05$ compared to pretreatment volume

at the distal one-third of the radius did not change significantly in either treatment group.

Following therapy, menses returned after 11.4 ± 3.2 weeks (mean ± standard error) following cessation of SC therapy and after 6.5 ± 1.8 weeks following completion of IN treatment. Unfortunately, uterine volume increased to near pretreatment size by 4 months following therapy in the SC group. Thus, the effects of leuprolide acetate on uterine size and menstruation appear to be temporary as noted by other investigators [9-12,14].

Hot flashes were experienced by all SC patients but only 4 of 7 IN patients were troubled by vasomotor instability. All patients reported that the intensity of hot flashes decreased with increasing duration of therapy.

SUBCUTANEOUS LEUPROLIDE ACETATE WITH OR WITHOUT MEDROXY-PROGESTERONE ACETATE IN THE TREATMENT OF LEIOMYOMATA UTERI

The above described study clearly demonstrated that SC leuprolide was more effective in decreasing uterine volume, inducing amenorrhea, and causing temporary resolution of fibroid-related symptoms than was IN leuprolide. Subcutaneously administered leuprolide also caused profound hypoestrogenism which was associated with development of hot flashes. A second study [10] was therefore designed in an attempt to eliminate or reduce the occurrence of hot flashes in women treated with SC leuprolide.

Medroxyprogesterone acetate (MPA) 20 mg orally each day has been reported to eliminate 74% of vasomotor flushes in postmenopausal women [16]. In our second study, premenopausal women were treated with SC leuprolide acetate and randomized to receive either MPA 20 mg orally each day, or placebo tablets. Sixteen women enrolled and seven received leuprolide acetate plus placebo (group A); nine received leuprolide acetate plus MPA

(group B). Both groups were treated for 24 weeks. Presenting
symptoms were similar to those in the first study.
     All patients in both groups completed the 24 weeks treatment
period. All patients in group A had resolution of their
presenting symptoms; only five of nine patients in group B
experienced resolution. In group A, serum E_2 concentrations
fell from a pretreatment mid-luteal phase baseline of 178 pg/ml to
20 pg/ml by 4 weeks of therapy and remained in the postmenopausal
range throughout treatment. A similar degree of hypoestrogenism
was achieved in group B, with E_2 falling from 194 pg/ml prior to
therapy to 28 pg/ml by 4 weeks and remaining in the postmenopausal
range for the duration of therapy. There were no significant
differences in estradiol concentrations between the 2 groups at
any treatment week.
     In group A, uterine volume decreased from 601 ± 62 cm^3
prior to therapy to 388 ± 75 cm^3 by 8 weeks (p<0.05) and to 307
± 45 cm^3 at 12 weeks of therapy (p<0.01) (Table 3). Only

Table 3. Uterine volume (cm^3) in women treated with subcutaneous
leuprolide plus placebo versus subcutaneous leuprolide plus
medroxyprogesterone acetate (MPA)

	Leuprolide + Placebo n=7	Leuprolide + MPA n=9
Pretreatment	601 ± 62[a]	811 ± 174
4 weeks therapy	520 ± 111	821 ± 195
8 weeks therapy	388 ± 75[b]	720 ± 195
12 weeks therapy	307 ± 45[c]	738 ± 173
24 weeks therapy	294 ± 46[c]	688 ± 154

[a] Mean $\pm$ standard error
[b] p<0.05 compared to pretreatment volume
[c] p<0.01 compared to pretreatment volume

minimal further shrinkage to 294 ± 46 cm^3 was noted at 24 weeks
of therapy (p<0.01 versus baseline). In contrast, uterine volume
did not significantly decrease in group B at any treatment period
when compared to pretreatment volume. The mechanism of the
preventive action of MPA on leuprolide induced uterine regression
is not understood. It cannot be attributed to the degree of
estrogen suppression as this was similar in both groups. Perhaps
MPA or one of its metabolites induces myometrial growth thus
counteracting the expected effect of uterine shrinkage seen with a
profoundly hypoestrogenic state.
     Hemoglobin concentrations, hematocrits and serum iron
concentrations increased significantly in both groups at 24 weeks

of therapy. This was attributed to amenorrhea induced in both groups (except for minimal vaginal spotting noted in 4 of 9 patients in group B).

Fasting serum cholesterol, high density lipoprotein (HDL) cholesterol, and triglyceride concentrations increased slightly but not significantly in both groups at 12 and 24 weeks of therapy when compared to pretreatment values. Total cholesterol/HDL cholesterol ratios, an index of cardiovascular disease risk, did not change during therapy.

Six of 7 patients in Group A experienced hot flashes whereas only 1 of 9 patients noted this symptom in Group B ($p < 0.01$, Fisher's exact test). This is consistent with the findings of Schiff et al [16] that MPA successfully reduces the incidence of hot flashes in postmenopausal women. Menses returned by 7 weeks in all patients in both groups. Uterine volume was not recorded in the follow-up period.

CONCLUSIONS

Subcutaneous leuprolide (0.5 mg) is more successful than IN leuprolide (0.8 mg bid) in inducing hypoestrogenism, amenorrhea, reduction in uterine volume and resolution of symptoms due to uterine leiomyomata. The effects of leuprolide are temporary. The per cent reduction in uterine volume is negatively correlated with serum E_2 concentration. The addition of oral MPA to SC leuprolide prevents uterine shrinkage. Subcutaneous leuprolide, with or without MPA, may induce significant increases in hemoglobin concentration, hematocrit, and serum iron concentration, presumably by stopping menstruation. This may be important in the treatment of anemic women with leiomyomata prior to surgical therapy as pre-operative anemia increases the likelihood of blood transfusions in women undergoing hysterectomy or myomectomy [17].

Oral MPA when added to SC leuprolide decreases the incidence of hot flashes. Treatment with SC leuprolide, with or without MPA, for 24 weeks does not appear to adversely effect the serum lipid profile.

REFERENCES

1.   Robbins, SL, and Cortran RS (1979). Leiomyomata (fibromyoma). In "The Pathogenic Basis of Disease". p.1271. (Philadelphia: WB Sanders Co)
2.   Novak, ER, and Woodruff, JD (1979). Myoma and other benign tumors of the uterus. In "Gynecologic and Obstetric Pathology". p.260. (Philadelphia: WB Sanders Co)
3.   Babaknia, A, Rock, JA, and Jones HW (1978). Pregnancy success following abdominal myomectomy for infertility. Fertil Steril, 30, 644
4.   Ingersoll, FM (1963). Fertility following myomectomy. Fertil Steril, 14, 596

5.   Hunt, JE, and Wallach, EE (1974). Uterine factors in infertility-an overview. Clin Obstet Gynecol, 17, 44

6.   Esterday, CL, Grimes, DA, and Riggs, JA (1983). Hysterectomy in the United States. Obstet Gynecol, 62, 203

7.   Lipshultz, A (1942). Experimental fibroids and the antifibromatogenic action of steroid hormones. JAMA, 120, 173

8.   Nelson, WO, (1937). Endometrial and myometrial changes including fibromyomatous nodules induced in the guinea pig by oestrogen. Anat Rec, 68, 99

9.   Friedman, AJ, Barbieri, RL, Benaceraff, BR, and Schiff, I (1987). Treatment of leiomyomata with intranasal or subcutaneous leuprolide, a gonadotropin releasing-hormone agonist. Fertil Steril, 48, 560

10.   Friedman, AJ, Barbieri, RL, Doubilet, PM, Fine, C, and Schiff, I (1988). A randomized, double-blind trial of a gonadotropin releasing-hormone agonist (leuprolide) with or without medroxyprogesterone acetate in the treatment of leiomyomata uteri. Fertil Steril (in press)

11.   Healy, DL, Lawson, SR, Abbott, M, Baird, DT, and Fraser, HM (1986). Toward removing uterine fibroids without surgery: Subcutaneous infusion of a luteinizing hormne-releasing hormone agonist commencing in the luteal phase. J Clin Endocrinol Metab, 63, 619

12.   Coddington, CC, Collins, RL, Shawker, TH, Anderson, R, Loriaux, DL, and Winkel, CA (1986). Long-acting gonadotropin hormone-releasing hormone analog used to treat uteri. Fertil Steril, 45, 624

13.   Filicore, M, Hall, DA, Loughlin, JA, Rivier, J, Vale, W, and Crowley WF (1983). A conservative approach to the management of uterine leiomyoma: Pituitary desensitization by a luteinizing hormone-releasing hormone analogue. Am J Obstet Gynecol, 146, 726

14.   Maheux, R, Guilloteau, C, Lemay, A, Bastide, A, and Fazekas AIA (1985). Luteinizing hormone-releasing hormone agonist and uterine leiomyoma: A pilot study. Am J Obstet Gynecol, 152, 1034

15.   Anik, ST, McRae, G, Nerenberg, C, Worden, A, Foreman, J, Jwang J-Y, Kushinsky, S, Jones, RE and Vickery, B (1984). Nasal absorption of nafarelin acetate, the decapeptide [D-Nal(2)6]-LHRH, in rhesus monkey I. J Pharm Sci, 23, 684

16.   Schiff, I, Tulchinsky, D, Cramer, D, and Ryan, KJ (1980). Oral medroxyprogesterone in the treatment of postmenopausal symptoms. JAMA, 244, 1443

17.   Mintz, PD and Sullivan, MF (1985). Preoperative crossmatch ordering and blood use in elective hysterectomy. Obstet Gynecol, 65, 389

4

RELEVANCE OF AN LHRH AGONIST TO THE TREATMENT OF UTERINE FIBROMYOMAS

J. COHEN and **D. ELIA**
Clinique Marignan, 3 rue Marignan, 75008 Paris, France

INTRODUCTION

Uterine fibromyomas are among the most common benign pelvic tumours in women. They are linked with a number of problems which, most often, without being serious in themselves or in isolation, make up a clinical picture which can be functionally bothersome (abdominal discomfort and painful heaviness, menorrhagia and, sometimes, metrorrhagia with clots and pain, hypofertility and/or a possible risk of haemorrhagic complications during delivery or immediately post partum).
Up to now, the recommended treatments were, namely, no intervention if the fibroma does not cause evident problems, prescription of a progestational agent for 20 days during each menstrual cycle or, ultimately, surgery, which, depending on circumstances, may be limited simply to ablation of any existing myoma or myomas, or involve hysterectomy, with or without preservation of the ovaries. Progestational treatment brings about cessation or diminution of menometrorrhagia but does not reduce myomal volume.
It is a fact that the menopause always results in a reduction in fibromyomal size and in disappearance of the problems caused by fibromyomas. Various studies [1,2] have also shown that uterine fibromatous tissue is richer in oestrogen receptors than healthy uterine tissue. This supports the idea that fibromyomas are oestrogen-dependent and that a reduction in this hormone could be beneficial in the treatment of this complaint.
A therapeutic possibility of this kind is now offered by LHRH agonists, which have recently become available in two indications for which a hormonosuppressive effect is sought, prostatic cancer and precocious puberty.
It is known that, after an initial brief stimulation phase, these agents act by a desensitization at the level of the pituitary receptors, and that they cause a decline in the levels of the two gonadotrophins, FSH and LH. Ten to 15 days after they have begun to be administered, there is onset of a hypogonadotrophic state of hypogonadism, characterized biologically by reduced levels of oestradiol or testosterone,

below what is termed the castration threshold, and this effect continues for as long as treatment continues.

In the last one or two years, various investigators have studied LHRH agonists in small groups of patients with uterine fibromyomas, and have detailed in various publications progress recorded in relation to reduction in uterine volume (Table 1), the reduction being on average between 50 and 55%, depending on the agonist used (apart from a gain in volume with leuprolide as a nasal spray [3]).

Table 1. Results of previously published studies on changes in uterine volume

Author [ref]	Year	Product	Route	Duration	No. of Cases	Percentage Change in Uterine Volume
Coddington [5]	1986	Buserelin	SC	6 months	6	-57
Perl [6]	1987	D-Trp[6] LHRH	SC	3 months	10	-42.5
West [7]	1987	Zoladex	Depot	6 months	13	-55
Maheux [8]	1987	Buserelin	Spray	6 months	9	-71
Friedman [3]	1987	Leuprolide	Spray	6 months	7	+10
			SC	6 months	7	-53

It therefore seemed to us interesting to assess the therapeutic possibilities of LHRH agonists in this indication, particularly since the previous studies had not indicated any toxicity, and had even eliminated the risk, significant in our view, of a reduction in bone mineral reserves, the incidence and importance of which in postmenopausal women are now better known. The study of Friedman et al. [3] is reassuring in this connection. It relates to women who were still young (premenopausal), all of whom were treated for a period of six months.

To carry out the present study, we chose [D-Trp[6]]LHRH (tryptorelin), which has the advantage of being capable of being administered intramuscularly once a month, thanks to the existence of a sustained-release dosage form containing 3.75 mg of active principle, which allows liberation of a theoretical dose of 100 μg/day for 30 days into the body. Studies in man have shown that, after an initial phase of release of active principle present on the surface of the microcapsules, there is a phase of regular release of [D-Trp[6]]LHRH, the mean equilibrium rate of which is 46.6 ± 7.1 μg/day, with a bioavailability of about 53% at one month, which is perfectly satisfactory. In addition, it has now been established that, even after prolonged LHRH agonist treatment, for six months or more, the effect of the agent stops once it has disappeared from the body, hormonal levels reverting to normal values. In the case of [D-Trp^6]LHRH, it has been confirmed in women who have not yet gone through the menopause that normal, regular menstruation recurs on average 87 days after the final administration of a sustained release form [4].

We report below results obtained in 14 patients with one or more uterine fibromyoma, whom we treated for a period of six months with [D-Trp^6]LHRH.

MATERIAL AND METHODS

Fourteen women, who were premenopausal and, therefore, menstruating regularly, each of whom had one or more uterine fibromyoma with uteri increased in volume (by 100 to 978 cm^3) were enrolled into this study and monitored under over supervision, both clinically and echographically. Their ages ranged from 24 to 51 years. Seven had had no children, 2 had 1 child and 5 had 2 children.

These 14 patients were fully informed of their participation in a therapeutic trial involving certain constraints as regards monitoring, and that they would be given a monthly injection of a drug which was known but which was still under trial in this indication. All gave their agreement to treatment, particularly since most were troubled in daily life by their fibroma(s) and had not so far been adequately relieved by the various treatments undertaken.

The problems had in fact often been increasing for several months and diagnoses of fibromyomas had been made. Eight complained of discomfort and abdominal pain of severe nature between periods, the latter being particularly troublesome and painful in five cases. Eight patients also complained of menometrorrhagias with significant hypermenorrhoea in four cases, more moderate in the other four.

Uterine volume was initially assessed clinically by gynaecological examination, repeated whenever monitoring took place. However, for its quantitative evaluation, we took account only of measurements made using ultrasonography, always making use of the same echographists, asking them to indicate as precisely as possible the three main dimensions of the uterine body, its breadth (measured between the two horns), its length (or uterine height) and, lastly, its thickness (or anteroposterior diameter). From these three parameters, we calculated the uterine volume, using the formula $4/3\pi$ R1 x R2 x R3, where R1, R2 and R3 correspond to half of the dimensions mentioned above.

Thus each of our patients was the subject of such a determination before the start of therapy, three months later, and finally, six months later, at the end of the trial. Several patients were also the subjects of intermediate checks, one patient having undergone monthly checking throughout the six months of the study.

Before treatment began, the uterine volume was between 100 cm^3 for the smallest and 678 cm^3 for the largest, with a mean value of 321 ± 77 cm^3. Echographic monitoring also allowed localization and measurement of the various myomas (of a size equal to or greater than 15 mm). Patients with intracavitary myomas, with myomas undergoing changes in shape or with necrobiosis, and with ovarian cysts, and patients who were pregnant were excluded. Patients who had undergone radiological or surgical castration and patients with any other serious or neoplastic disease were also excluded.

Twenty-nine myomas were initially identified (Table 2).

Table 2. Relative incidence of myomas

Number of Myomas	Incidence
1	6 cases
2	3 cases
3	4 cases
5	1 case

In each patient, the investigations were completed by a systematic screening smear and hysterography, unless these examinations had recently been carried out.

A biological investigation was also undertaken before the start of the trial, with the determinations necessitated by the condition of each patient and needed to assess tolerance, which we wished to verify in some cases. From the hormonal point of view, we performed investigations relating mainly to determination of oestradiol, FSH and LH, supplemented by determinations of prolactin and progesterone. The mean hormonal levels before treatment were as shown in Table 3.

Table 3. Pretreatment hormone levels

Hormone	Mean Value (pg/ml)[*]
oestradiol	218 ± 49
FSH	4.22 ± 1.98 UI/l (9)
LH	1.86 ± 0.85 UI/l (8)

[*]Number of subjects

It was possible to repeat these checks in some patients at the third or sixth month after the start of treatment. [D-Trp[6]]LHRH was administered every 28 days. Fourteen patients were treated. Twelve received 6 injections of [D-Trp[6]]LHRH at the rate of one every 28 or 30 days. Of the 2 others, 1 received 3 injections and the other 4. They were not seen after the 3 month check, having left for the provinces. We deliberately avoided choosing a particular day within the menstrual cycle for carrying out the first injection, since the risk of the patient becoming pregnant seemed to us to be much reduced. Obviously, we abstained during the study from all concomitant therapy. Even products capable of altering the degree of menorrhagia were prohibited. Patients with IUDs were allowed to retain them. As far as hot flushes during treatment were concerned, we abstained voluntarily from any prescription whenever possible.

RESULTS

The results of the six-month trial administration are presented in Table 4.

In summary, all clinical symptoms consistent with the presence of one or more fibromyoma became progressively less marked and disappeared completely in the first three months of treatment. Thus feelings of discomfort or abdominal heaviness, experienced by eight women before treatment, were notified in only two cases in the third month, and by no patient thereafter. Dysmenorrhoea, present in five cases, completely disappeared in the first two months. Menometrorrhagia was also very rapidly affected from the first month on (persisting at the third month in only one patient), giving place to amenorrhoea, obtained from the first month in one case, before the end of the second month in seven cases and before the end of the third month in six cases, the differences probably being related to the time in the menstrual cycle at which the first injection was given. Review of the echographic uterine measurements demonstrates objectively the effect of [D-Trp[6]]LHRH. Before treatment, the mean uterine volume determined for all 14 patients was 321 ± 77 cm^3. Half-way through treatment, i.e. three months later, it had altered, for the same number of patients, to 155 ± 29 cm^3, (a reduction of 52%). At the end of treatment, it had fallen again, from 146 ± 28 cm^3 (the mean determined at the third month for the 12 patients who completed the full six-month study), to 112 ± 22 cm^3. This was less than that noted in the course of the first three months, but still progressive (Fig. 1).

Overall, the reduction of uterine volume obtained through this medical treatment, determined in the 12 patients whom it was possible to monitor echographically from the start of treatment to its termination, was 64%.

The reductions in the number of myomas and in their sizes was also monitored. On average, myomal size fell by 27%, regression being obtained in 8 patients and total disappearance in 2 patients. An increase in size was obtained in only 1 case, and

Table 4. Main characteristics of the patients in the trial. Results relating to uterine volume and myomas observed.

Pat.	Age (Y)	No. of Children	Symptoms Before Treatment	Uterine Volume cm³ Before	Uterine Volume cm³ After	Reduction (%)	Nos. and Sizes of Myomas Before	Nos. and Sizes of Myomas After	Response
1	24	0	Dysmenorrhoea, moderate menometrorrhagia	252	101	60	1, 53	0	Complete
2	39	2	Moderate menometrorrhagia	166	97	42	2, 32, 20	2, 18, 60	Complete
3	37	0	Discomfort, abdominal pains, dysmenorrhoea moderate meno-metrorrhagia	143	106 (M3) NR* M6	37 (M3) NR M6	5, 31, 27, 25	5, 28, 22, 21, 18, NR	Complete (M3)
4	39	1	Discomfort, abdominal pains	124	56	54.5	1, 23	1, 15	Complete
5	45	1	Substantial menometrorrhagia	248	102	59	3, 30, 12, 11	3, 28, 10, 12	Complete
6	45	2	Discomfort, abdominal pains, moderate menometrorrhagia	586	298 (M3) NR M6	49 (M3) NR M6	3, 11, 37, 55	3, 11, 35, 45, NR M6	Complete (M3)
7	47	0	Dysmenorrhoea moderate metrorrhagia	344	128	63	1, 55	1, 25	Complete
8	51	0	Discomfort, abdominal pains	880	183	79	3, 58, 36, 51	3, 49, 25, 36	Complete

*NR = non-review.

Table 4. (Continued) Main characteristics of the patients in the trial. Results relating to uterine volume and myomas observed.

Pat.	Age (Y)	No. of Children	Symptoms Before Treatment	Uterine Volume cm³		Reduction (%)	Nos. and Sizes of Myomas		Response
				Before	After		Before	After	
9	42	2	Discomfort, abdominal pains, moderate metrorrhagia	133	61	54	1 22	1 28	Partial (myomal growth)
10	48	0	Discomfort, abdominal pains, substantial menometrorrhagia	978	330	66	1 70	1 65	Complete
11	38	0		251	58	77	3 40, 40, 30	3 30, 22, 18	Complete
12	27	2		100	51	49	2 26, 35	0 -	Complete
13	42	2	Discomfort, abdominal pains, dysmenorrhoea, substantial menometrorrhagia	173	98	43	2 30, 23	2 24, 21	Complete
14	46	0	Discomfort, abdominal pains, substantial menometrorrhagia	115	81	30	1 55	1 48	Complete

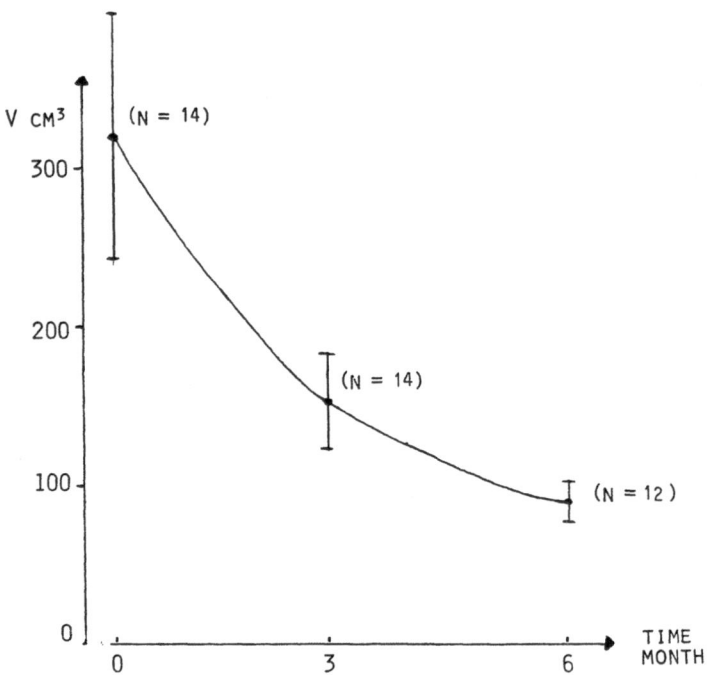

FIGURE 1   Decline in uterine volume

nonuniform alteration in another patient, who had 3 myomas. Two
regressed, the third increased in size.
      From the biological and, in particular, hormonal point of
view, the checks made confirmed the reductions in levels of
oestradiol, FSH and LH. In 5 patients, we repeated biological/
hormonal determinations at the end of the first month to be
certain that castration was effective. The following mean values
were obtained: Oestradiol 33 ± 16.2 pg/ml, FSH 2.56 ± 1.36 UI/l,
LH 1.4 ± 0.54 UI/l.
      In addition, we monitored the plasma level of estradiol,
which fell from 218 ± 49 pg/ml before treatment to 37.2 ±
7.8 pg/ml at the third month and to 21.6 ± 2.9 pg/ml at the end of
treatment.

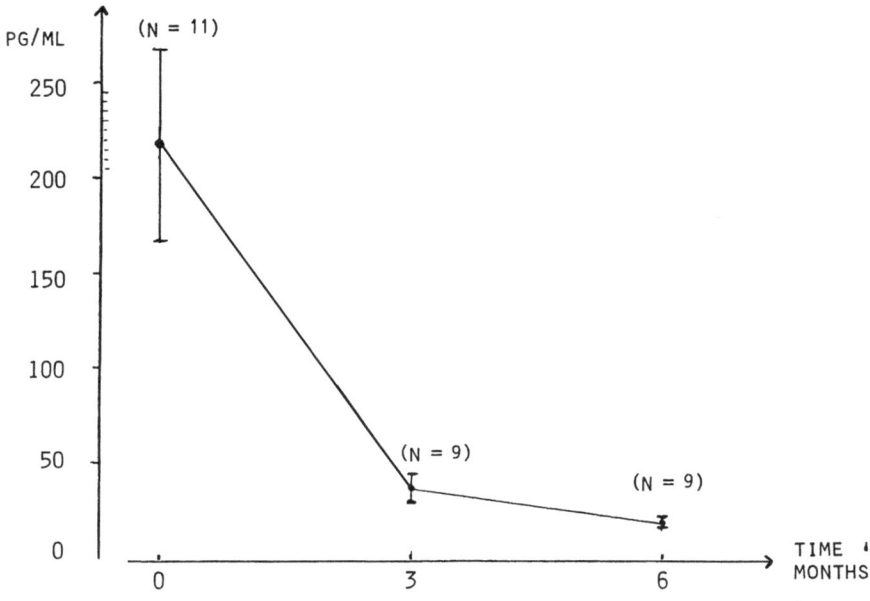

FIGURE 2   Reduction in plasma oestradiol levels

          Figure 2 shows the alteration in blood oestradiol levels.
It may be compared with Figure 1. By doing so, the correlation
which exists between the regression in uterine volume, myomal size
and the reduction in levels of this hormone may be seen.

TOLERANCE

Examination of tolerance also played an important part in our
study. It is known that any treatment with an LHRH agonist
results in a hypo-oestrogenic state which can be badly tolerated
by young women. In this connection, all of our patients were the
subjects of very regular monitoring, to collect their complaints
and assess their importance.
          Preparation of the injections and their administration
caused no problems once sufficient, minimal experience had been
gained.

41

Of the 79 injections undertaken, a small, painful zone of induration around the injection site was exhibited by only one patient following the first administration, for several days. All of the other injections were perfectly absorbed and no local phenomena were notified.

General tolerance was investigated by systematically questioning each patient during each consultation, going through a standard list of possible side effects. This procedure undoubtedly allowed more complaints to be noted than the patients would have described spontaneously, and, although four patients, i.e. one fourth of those treated, reported no problems during the six months of the trial, 10 patients reported hot flushes. This symptom is, therefore, common, and has been reported in all studies on the use of LHRH agonists in premenopausal women. It is, in any case, a reflection, or the almost inevitable consequence of the therapeutic mode of action of such drugs.

In our study, these hot flushes appeared most often at the end of the first month. They predominated at night or in the morning and varied in intensity, depending on the day. Although sometimes disagreeable, they always remained tolerable, and began to diminish, in general, three to four months after the start of treatment. They also disappeared completely in two patients before the study ended. None of the women asked for treatment to be stopped for this reason.

Also in direct relationship to the hypo-oestrogenicity produced by the treatment, one patient complained of vaginal dryness and another of dyspareunia for a limited period, but the latter patient was suffering at the same time from cystitis. One patient reported a slight recurrence of headaches.

We also had 3 patients who occasionally reported a state of fatigue and/or lassitude, and 2 who exhibited a depressive phase, transient and minor in one case, and more severe in the other case, necessitating prescription of appropriate treatment for a brief period. However, it was possible to continue treatment with [D-Trp^6]LHRH for the full term.

Finally, 2 patients alleged that there were marked reductions in the volumes of their breasts, which was not necessarily disadvantageous, especially in a case of associated mastopathy, and four patients reported occurrence of slight spotting during the first weeks of treatment.

DISCUSSION

As regards the results, the percentage regression observed on [D-Trp^6]LHRH was compared with the percentages already published on this topic (Table 3). From this, it is evident that the ultimate results vary according to the investigator.

Table 5. Changes in uterine volume with different LHRH agonists

Investigator [ref]	Day 0	M6	Change (%)	Subsequent Change
Coddington [5] (busereline SC)	539 ± 394	229 ± 145	−57	Results unchanged for next 3 to 7 months
West [7] (zoladex depot)	360 ± 225	162 ± 100	−55	367 ± 288 (+126%) 4 months later
Friedman [3] (leuprolide SC)	368 ± 60	172 ± 49	−53	296 ± 104 (+72%) 4 months later
Cohen & Elia* [D-Trp^6]LHRH	314 ± 86	112 ± 22	−64	

*present study

These results are better than with progestagens. They cannot be compared with myomectomy and hysterectomy, which remove the myomas and obviously retain their specific indications. However, myomectomy sometimes leads to adhesions and to recurrences, and hysterectomy has psychological and physiological sequelae, and morbidity.

As regards tolerance, [D-Trp^6]LHRH has no particularly harmful side effect and, as a general rule, has proved to be well tolerated and accepted in young, premenopausal women. Its sole inconvenience is that it creates a hypo-oestrogenic state, as a direct consequence of its mode of action and, therefore, the hot flushes with mood problems which it can cause are more or less inevitable.

Overall, [D-Trp^6]LHRH is a completely efficacious treatment for uterine fibromyomas. Its effect is rapid (from the second month), perceptible to both the patient (disappearance of bleeding) and the practitioner (reduction in uterine volume). It can be objectively demonstrated by echography (regression of myomas and of uterine volume). It is an easy and convenient treatment, requiring only once a month administration. Its optimum duration seems to us to be four to six months. Its tolerance is satisfactory despite the relative discomfort caused by the hot flushes. Its fairly high cost must be compared with the advantages it can offer. However, at present, it is too soon to judge its long-term effect, and we are therefore continuing regularly monitoring of our patients.

This treatment therefore has numerous advantages and could take a place in the treatment of uterine fibromyomas in accordance with the following schedule: It should be reserved for symptomatic myomas and should not replace surgery in cases of complications, severe compression or myomas which are substantial and excessive in volume. When the menopause is not near, treatment is prescribed for six months. If a reduction in myomal volume is obtained, patients are monitored clinically. If there is no recurrence, there is no treatment. If there is recurrence, operation should be undertaken. If recurrence is late, repetition of treatment may be considered. When the menopause is near, if there has been no recurrence the patient is monitored and prescription of a sequential, natural, low-dose oestrogen-progestogen treatment may be considered. If myomas and symptoms have recurred, recourse to surgery is necessary.

This treatment may also be envisaged prior to surgery, allowing a reduction in size of myoma and, perhaps, simplifying their removal. Other studies will be needed to determine whether or not this treatment can avoid the need for myomectomy in cases of sterility associated with the presence of myomas.

REFERENCES

1. Pollow, K. Geilfuss, J, Rowuoi, E and Pollow, B (1978). Estrogen and progesterone-binding proteins in normal human myometrium and leiomyoma tissue. J Clin Chem Biochem, 16, 503
2. Wilson, EA, Ynag, F and Rees, ED (1980). Estradiol and progesterone binding in uterine leimoyomata and in normal uterine tissues. Obstet Gynecol, 55, 20
3. Friedman, AJ, Barhieri, RI, Benacerraf, BR, and Schiff, I (1987). Treatment of leiomyomata with intranasal or subcutaneous leuprolide, a gonadotropin-releasing hormone agonist. Fertil Steril, 48, 560
4. Sureau, C and Zorn, JR. Essai therapeutique du [D-Trp^6]LHRH au cours de l'endometriose. (personal communication)
5. Coddington, CC, Collins, RL, Shawker, TH, Anderson, R, Leplay, DL and Winkel, CA (1986). Long-acting gonadotropin hormone-releasing hormone analog used in treat uteri. Fertil Steril, 5, 621
6. Perl, V, Leal, O, Marquez, J, Zacharias, S, Schally, AV, Gomez-Lira, C and Comaru-Schally, AM (1987). Treatment of leimyomata uteri with [D-Trp^6]-luteinizing hormone-releasing horomone. Fertil Steril, 48, 383
7. West, CP, Williamson, J, Lumsden, MA, Baird, DT and Lawson, S (1987). Shrinkage of uterine fibroids during therapy with goserelin (zoladex): a luteinizing hormone-releasing hormone agonist administered as a monthly subcutaneous depot. Fertil Steril, 48, 45
8. Maheux, R, Lemay, A and Merat, P (1987). Use of intranasal luteinizing hormone-releasing hormone agonist in uterine leiomyomas. Fertil Steril, 47, 229

5

COMPARISON OF TREATMENT OF UTERINE LEIOMYOMATA WITH 3 DIFFERENT GnRH AGONISTIC ANALOGS

Z. BLUMENFELD, M. DIRNFIELD, D. BECK, H. ABRAMOVIC
and **J.M.BRANDES**
Department of Obstetrics and Gynecology, Rambam Medical Center,
Carmel Hospital, Technion, Israel Institute of Technology, Haifa,
Israel 31096

INTRODUCTION

Uterine leiomyomata are the most common solid tumor of the female genital tract and may cause heavy menometrorrhagia, pelvic pain or discomfort, infertility and habitual abortion [1]. Uterine myomectomy is not always feasible, and total hysterectomy may result from surgical attempts to treat leiomyomata in young women who are still interested in childbearing. Estrogens are known to play a key role in the development and enlargement of uterine leiomyomata. High levels of estrogen receptors have been found in this type of tumor and exogenous administration of synthetic estrogens may result in rapid increase in the size of uterine leiomyomata [2, 3]. Since virtually all uterine leiomyomata are benign [4, 5] attempts have been made to offer a conservative medical approach to the surgical alternative of hysterectomy. Moreover, the pregnancy rate following myomectomy is only 40% [6]. The success of this operation is inversely related to the size of the myomatous uterus at the time of surgery [6]. In 15% of patients having had surgical myomectomy recurrence will take place, two thirds necessitating a second surgery [6].

Due to these observations, the creation of a temporary hypo-estrogenic state in theory would be beneficial. Initial studies have demonstrated rapid regression to occur in most patients [1, 4-8] following pituitary desensitization by GnRH agonistic analogs.

To further evaluate the efficacy and side effects of this form of treatment, we have administered a monthly intramuscular (IM) injection of [D-Trp^6]GnRH (Decapeptyl, Ferring, FRG) in a microencapsulated form to 21 patients for 6 months and compared them to 12 other patients with uterine leiomyomata treated by daily nasal applications of either [D-Nal(2)^6]GnRH (Synarel®; nafarelin, Syntex, USA) or [D-Ser(tBu)^6,Pro^{9}NHEt]GnRH (buserelin, Hoechst, FRG).

MATERIALS AND METHODS

Twenty one women with symptomatic uterine leiomyomas were treated with a monthly injection of microencapsulated [D-Trp^6]-GnRH 3.2mg, for 6 months. Their ages ranged from 27 to 51 years. Ten patients were perimenopausal, 48-51 years old (y.o.), and 11 were still interested in fertility (27-43 y.o.). These 21 patients (Group A) were compared to 12 other patients treated by nasal application of either nafarelin, (Group B - 10 patients) or buserelin (Group C - 2 patients). All patients were treated for a period of 6 months; treatment beginning between the 2nd and the 5th day of the cycle. The ages of the patients in group B were 30-43 years and in group C, 49 and 53 years. Indications for treatment were menometrorrhagia, pelvic pain or discomfort, or infertility, associated with myomatous uteri of 9-18 weeks of pregnancy determined by pelvic examination and trans-vaginal sonography (TVS) (groups A,C), or by magnetic resonance imaging (MRI) (group B). Informed consent was obtained from all patients.
 Group B patients were treated for 6 months with nafarelin, (400μg twice daily), administered as a nasal spray. Group C patients were treated for 6 months with buserelin (400μg three times daily) administered as a nasal spray; after 3 months the dosage was decreased to 200μg three times daily. Blood samples were drawn in the early follicular phase in a control cycle prior to treatment and monthly during the study. Blood samples were assayed by RIA for gonadotropins (LH and FSH), 17-β-estradiol (E$_2$), testosterone (T), androstenedione (Δ4A; only in group B) and dehydroepiandrosterone sulfate (DHEA-S; only in group B). Patients were examined monthly and uterine size was recorded as compared to weeks of pregnancy. Endometrial biopsies were performed in 16 patients prior to and after treatment. Pelvic MRI was used to assess uterine and myoma size in group B [9] amd TVS or abdominal sonography was used in group A and group C patients, for uterine and myoma size measurements. MRI scans were performed prior to, at 3 and 6 months of treatment and TVS on every monthly visit. Uterine and myomata volumes were calculated by the formula for the volume of an ellipsoid sphere (π/6xaxbxc); a, b and c representing the length, width and depth, respectively. Statistical evaluations of data were made using a computerized analysis of variance (ANOVA) for repeated measurements [9].

RESULTS

All but 2 patients completed the treatment. One patient discontinued treatment due to failure to follow the protocol and the other due to depression. All patients, on all the 3 analogs, experienced hot flashes graded as moderate to severe, but in no case was it a reason for discontinuation of treatment. All the patients in group A became amenorrheic within 60 days and all but one in groups B and C became amenorrheic within 90 days. The pre-treatment endometrial biopsies demonstrated proliferative or secretory endometrium and were appropriate for the phase of the menstrual cycle. After 6 months of analog treatment the endometrial biopsies demonstrated inactive endometrium.

Estradiol concentrations decreased from follicular phase values (51±8.3pg/ml) before treatment to less than 20pg/ml in all groups at 3 months (p<0.001). Testosterone, Δ4A and DHEA-S concentrations did not change significantly during the analog treatment. Although LH and FSH concentrations decreased significantly by 3 and 6 months of treatment (p<0.01) they did not reach hypogonadotropic concentrations; they remained at the lower range for normal values (5-7mIU/ml).

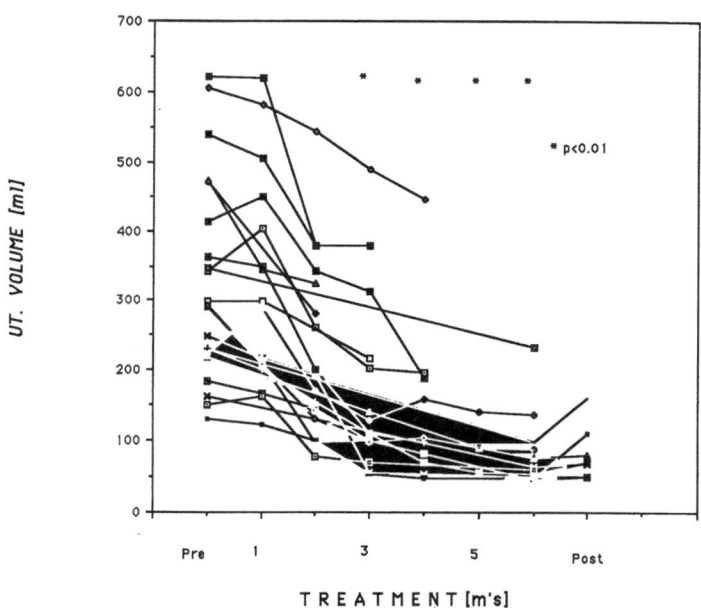

FIGURE 1 Uterine volume in 21 patients treated with monthly Decapeptyl-microencapsulated form

Uterine size decreased in all patients in group A by 24-80% as determined by TVS and pelvic examination (Figs 1 and 2). Most of the diminution in uterine volume was achieved within the first 3-4 months of treatment. In group B uterine size decreased, by pelvic examination, in 8 of 11 patients. The mean percent decrease in uterine volume was 51±10% in group A and 57±7% in group B by 7 months of treatment. The mean decrease in volume of the largest myoma was 47±9%.

The individual decrease in uterine or leiomyomata volumes was very variable. The amount of decrease in uterine volume ranged from 24 to 80% in group A and from 29-84% in groups B and C. Leiomyomata volumes decreased by 7-98%. Figs 3-5 illustrate

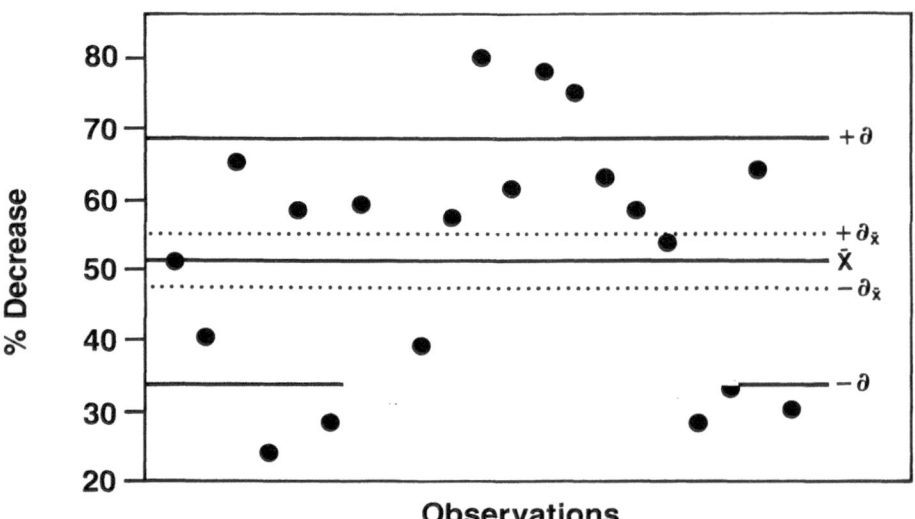

FIGURE 2 Scattergram of percentage % decrease in uterine volume in 21 patients after 6 months of decapeptyl treatment

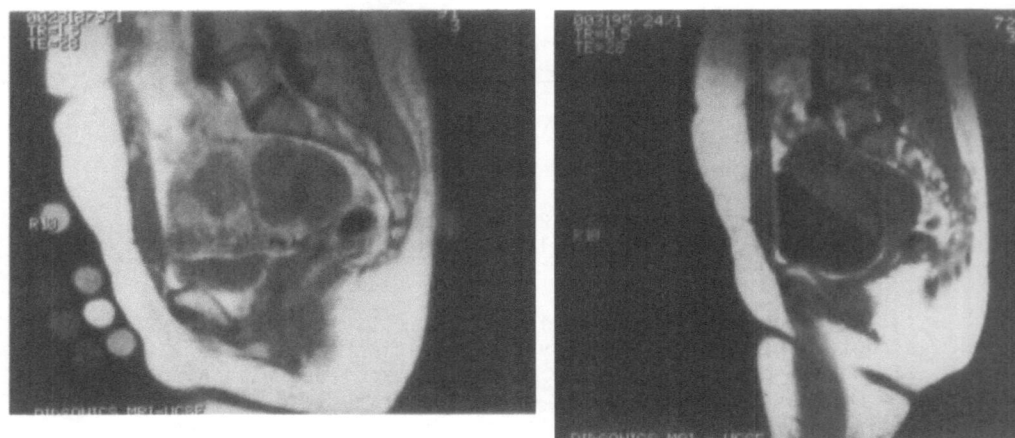

FIGURE 3 Uterine MRI before (left) and after (right) 3 months of nafarelin treatment

respresentative MRI and ultrasound scans of uteri before and after
3 months of agonist therapy. Six of the patients underwent
myomectomy while receiving decapeptyl or nafarelin. In all cases,
surgery was easily performed with reduced bleeding as compared to
myomectomy in untreated patients. The myometrium overlying the
myomata was thinner and less vascular than in untreated
premenopausal patients. After discontinuation of treatment
uterine volume increased in all premenopausal patients within 6
months of follow-up. However, in 4 patients over the
perimenopausal age vaginal bleeding did not recur after treatment
was discontinued; their uteri remained small and the hot flashes
continued. Hormonal evaluations were diagnostic of menopause.
All the other patients returned to menstruation within 2 months of
discontinuation of agonist treatment.

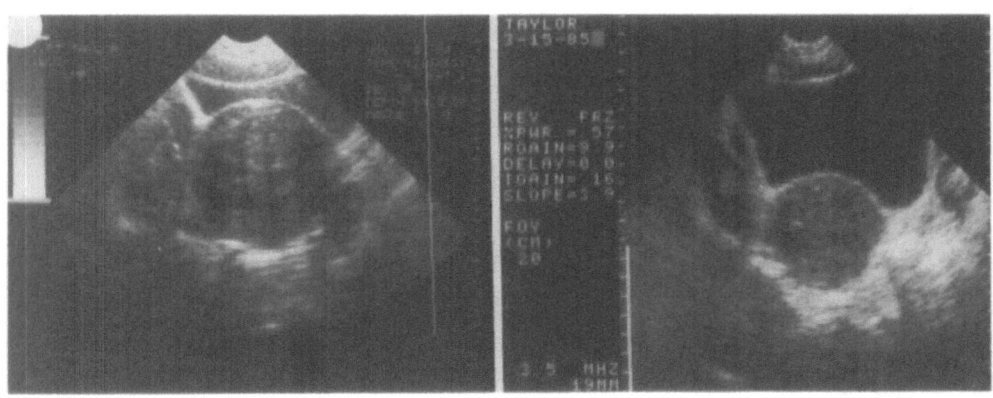

FIGURE 4   Uterine ultrasound before (left) and after (right) 3
       months of nasal nafarelin treatment

In one patient of childbearing age the pretreatment
hystero-salpingography (HSG) has shown bilateral cornual
obstruction. This patient underwent left salpingo-oophorectomy as
a child due to torsion of ovarian cyst. No other information was
available about the past surgery, which was performed in another
country. However, after completing 6 months of decapeptyl
treatment the uterine size decreased from the equivalent of 15
weeks of pregnancy to the size of a 9 weeks pregnant uterus and
the post treatment HSG has demonstrated patent right fallopian
tube with normal spillage of contrast solution.
In group B patients, quantitative computerized tomography
(QCT) of the lumbar vertebrae demonstrated a decrease in bone

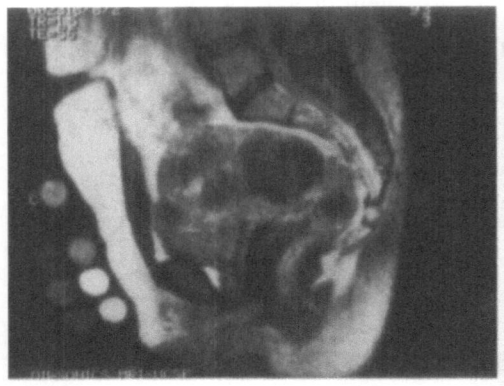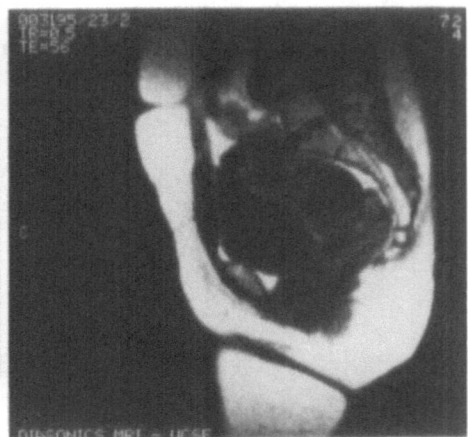

FIGURE 5   Uterine MRI before (left) and after (right) 3 months of
    nafarelin treatment

mineral content after 6 months of treatment of about 11%.
Although the value for estimated mineral content did not reach
values compatible with clinical osteoporosis (120mg/cc) the change
was statistically significant. Repeat QCT 6 months after
treatment was discontinued demonstrated return to almost
pre-treatment values.

DISCUSSION

All 3 analogs, decapeptyl, nafarelin and buserelin induced
significant hypoestrogenism, and amenorrhea in the treated
patients. Pelvic pain and discomfort were ameliorated and anemia
was abolished in all patients who suffered from these symptoms
prior to treatment. No significant changes in effect could be
detected between the different analogs used in this study.
Magnetic resonance imaging and TVS were both effective in
measuring uterine and leiomyomata size.

    As has been reported [4-8], the decrease in uterine and
leiomyomata volumes was very variable, 7-95%. Currently, there is
no accurate method to predict which patient will respond.
However, since most of the diminution in uterine size occurred
within the first 3-5 months of treatment, it may be more
effective, in terms of cost: effect ratio to spread 6 months of

agonist treatment over 9-10 months; i.e. to stop treatment after 3 months and repeat an additional course of 3 months treatment, if necessary, after 3 months without treatment.

As has been found previously [4-8], myomectomy was more easily performed after analog treatment, with minimal blood loss. This may possibly improve fertility after myomectomy since infertility and adhesion formation after myomectomy seem directly correlated to uterine and myomata sizes at the time of surgery, and to the amount of bleeding, respectively [6].

An hypoestrogenic state was achieved under all analog treatments. Whereas E_2 levels decreased to menopausal levels, radioimmunometric LH and FSH levels decreased significantly but remained above hypogonadotropic levels.

Finally, although no significant difference in the effect of the 3 different analogs was detected, patient compliance was better in the once monthly injection of the microencapsulated preparation group than in the nasal application groups.

Whereas the GnRH-analog treatment seems a temporary adjunct to myomectomy in the childbearing age, it may serve as a definitive treatment and replace surgery (hysterectomy) in the perimenopausal group. The 4 patients entering menopause immediately after completing the 6 months treatment period support this belief. Additional experience is needed to substantiate this treatment.

ACKNOWLEDGEMENTS

The assistance of Drs. Janice L. Andreyko, Scott E. Monroe and Robert B. Jaffe from the Reproductive Endocrinology Center, Dept. Ob/Gyn and Reproductive Sciences at Univ. California, San Francisco, and of Dr. Milan Henzl, Syntex Research is gratefully acknowledged.

REFERENCES

1.   Filicori, M, Hall, DA, Laughlin, JS, Rivier, J, Vale, W and Crowley, WF (1983). A conservative approach to the management of uterine leiomyoma: Pituitary desensitization by a luteinizing hormone releasing hormone analogue. Am J Obstet Gynecol, 147, 726
2.   Wilson, EA, Yang, F and Rees, ED (1980). Estradiol and progesterone binding in uterine leiomyomata and in normal uterine tissues. Obstet Gynecol, 55, 20
3.   Tamaya, T, Fujimoto, J and Okada, H (1985). Comparison of cellular levels of steroid receptors in uterine leiomyoma and myometrium. Acta Obstet Gynaecol Scand, 64, 307
4.   Maheux, R, Guilloteau, C, Lemay, A, Bastide, A and Fazekas, ATA (1985). Luteinizing hormone-releasing agonist and uterine leiomyoma: a pilot study. Am J Obstet Gynecol, 152, 1034
5.   Maheux, R, Lemay, A and Merat, P (1987). Use of intranasal luteinizing hormone-releasing hormone agonist in uterine leiomyomas. Fertil Steril, 47, 229

6.   Healy, DL, Lawson, SR, Abbott, M, Baird, DT and Fraser, HM (1986). Toward removing uterine fibroids without surgery: Subcutaneous infusion of a luteinizing hormone-releasing hormone agonist commencing in the luteal phase. J Clin Endocrinol Metab, 63, 619

7.   Coddington, CC, Collins, RL, Shawker, TH, Anderson, R, Loriaux, DL and Winkel, CA (1986). Long-acting gonadotropin hormone-releasing hormone analog used to treat uteri. Fertil Steril, 45, 624.

8.   van Leusden, HAIM (1986). Rapid reduction of uterine myomas after short-term treatment with microencapsulated D-Trp[6]-LHRH. Lancet, 1, 1213

9.   Winer, BJ (1971). Statistical principles in experimental design, p. 261. (New York: McGraw-Hill)

6

SEQUENTIAL BUSERELIN – MEDROXYPROGESTERONE ACETATE TREATMENT OF UTERINE LEIOMYOMATA

G. BENAGIANO, A. MORINI, A. ABBONDANTE, V. ALEANDRI, F. PICCINNO and D. SALA

First Institute of Obstetrics and Gynecology, University 'La Sapienza', Rome, Italy

INTRODUCTION

Estrogen dependency of uterine fibroids and an antagonistic effect of progesterone has been suspected for many years on the basis of clinical [1-5], as well as experimental observations [6-9]. In 1983 Filicori et al. [9] demonstrated that hypoestrogenism caused by chronic administration of a GnRH agonist produced a substantial reduction in the size of a large leiomyoma. Several investigators have since confirmed this finding [10-15].

Unresolved problems in the pharmacological treatment of fibroids include: the need to interrupt the administration of the analogue after a relatively short period of time (to avoid the negative consequence of hormonal deprivation), which entails the possibility of re-growth of the tumors [10, 11, 14]; the exact mechanism of action by which hypoestrogenism works and therefore an explanation of the lack of response which is occasionally observed; the role of steroid receptors in determining myomata development and therefore the possibility of blocking re-growth through receptor blockade.

To address these questions, our group has designed a series of studies, the preliminary results of which have already been presented [16-19].

The present report deals with the effect of sequentially administered buserelin and medroxyprogesterone acetate (MPA) on uterine size and fibroid re-growth.

MATERIALS AND METHODS

Clinical Material

A total of 45 women attending the out-patient clinic of the First Institute of Obstetrics and Gynecology of the University "La Sapienza" in Rome, in all of whom a clinical diagnosis of enlarged uteri (with or without echographically identifiable single or multiple leiomyomata) were selected for the study. The uteri ranged in volume between 47 and 770ml, and the identifiable myomata ranged between 3 and 302ml.

The subjects were divided into three groups: 5 women, who wished to become pregnant, were treated with buserelin for 6 months and then underwent surgery. The remaining 40 women were randomly assigned to two equal groups: the first received buserelin ([D-Ser(TBU)^{6}Pro^{9}NHEt]LHRH), subcutaneously at the daily dose of 1.5mg for one week, followed by 1.2mg intranasally until the end of the 28th week; they then served as controls during the following six months. The second group received buserelin for the same period of time followed by six months of treatment with MPA at the dose of 200 or 100mg per day for the first two months, 50mg per day for 2 additional months and 25mg per day for the last two months of treatment.

Ultrasound evaluation

The accuracy of ultrasound measurements was tested by comparing echographic determinations with those obtained after surgery, confirming that the systematic error in measurements does not exceed 20% [19]. All measurements were carried out by the same investigator using a real time Sonolayer-1 SAL 30A.

Morphological studies

In the five cases which were operated on at the end of six months of buserelin therapy, the myomatata were fixed and examined histologically, using standard techniques and under light microscopy.

RESULTS

Effect of buserelin

The administration of buserelin, over a period of six months to the 45 women, produced a substantial reduction of the size of the majority of the uteri. Giving a value of 100 to the volume of the organ before treatment, and of 0 to that of the average normal uterus (55ml), the reduction at 6 months was 54.6 ± 23.7%.

Four patients discontinued buserelin treatment before the scheduled six months. Two withdrew from the study because of allergic manifestations which were attributed to the medication; the other two were treated surgically because the uterus continued to grow in spite of the therapy.

Although the large variations in pre-treatment size make analysis difficult, the best responses were obtained with large uteri (800 to 400ml in volume). A total of 40 leiomyomata were identified by ultrasound in 36 of the 45 subjects. Following treatment, they decreased on the average by 61.3 ± 22.4%. Here again, the best results were obtained with large fibroids (200ml in volume).

In general, whenever a uterus showed a good response to the medication, a similar reduction was observed also in the myoma(s).

Effect of sequentially administered MPA

Following the six months of buserelin treatment, 18 of the 36 women were treated with MPA and the others served as controls.

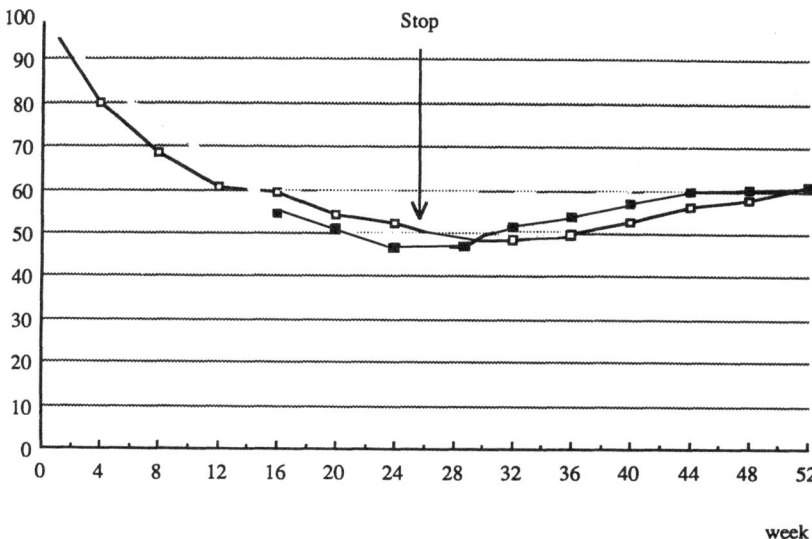

FIGURE 1   Percent decrease in the size of the uterus (A) and of identifiable fibromyomata (B) in two groups of 20 women following 24 weeks of therapy with buserelin.

On the average, after stopping buserelin medication, there was some re-growth of the size of the uterus both in the controls (Fig. 1) and in the MPA treated subjects (Fig. 2), with no statistically significant difference observed between the two groups.
A somewhat different picture was evident in the case of individual leiomyomata. Here, during the six months of MPA treatment no appreciable re-growth was observed in the fibroids, whereas some leiomyomata increased in size following discontinuation of buserelin administration alone. An analysis of variance showed that the difference between the two groups was statistically significant (p<0.01).

Changes in ultrasound appearance

During treatment with buserelin, the echo pattern of leiomyomata increased almost invariably as the volume decreased. In one case

55

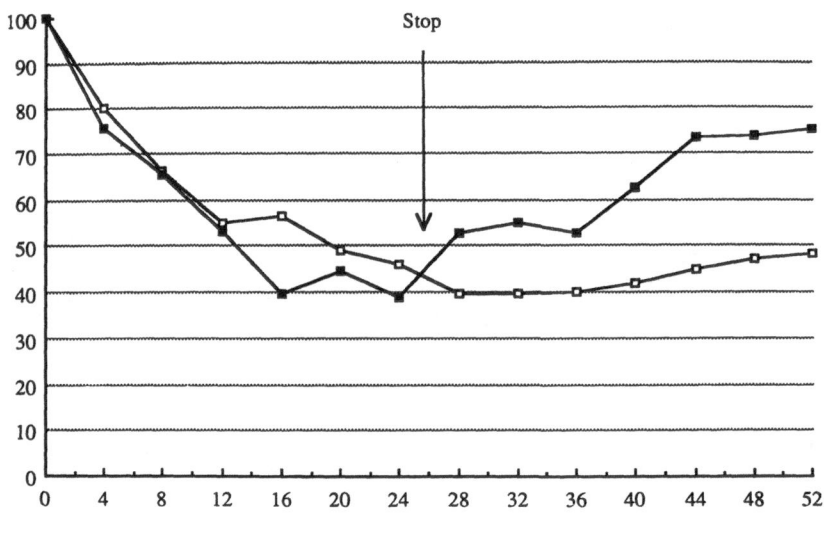

FIGURE 2 Group ■ was then followed without any additional
    medication and Group □ was treated with decreasing doses of
    MPA.

there was a complete echographic disappearance of the myoma.
    Occasionally, hypo-echoic areas were observed within the
confines of individual fibroids and these areas were the first to
show echographic modifications (Figs. 3 and 4).

Side effects

The incidence of those side effects commonly resulting from
estrogen deprivation produced by buserelin, was compared with that
observed in 50 healthy women in early menopause (Fig. 5). There
was a significant difference in the occurrence of sweating and
depression, which were much more frequent in post menopausal women
($p < 0.01$).
    Symptoms attributable to estrogen deficiency, completely
disappeared under MPA medication. However, when the daily MPA
dose was decreased below 100mg per day, however, the majority of
the patients experienced a degree of spotting.

Morphological studies

Histological evaluation of fibroid masses obtained from the 5
women in whom conservative surgery was carried out showed varying

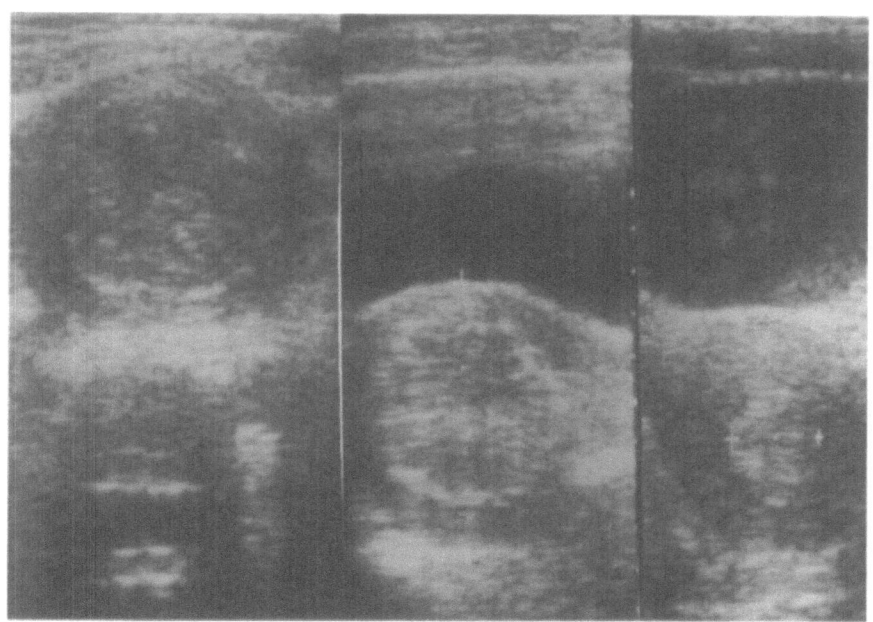

FIGURE 3   Changes in the ultrasound picture of a fibroid mass
            during therapy with buserelin showing the progressive
            shrinkage, with increased echogenicity of the mass, as
            treatment progresses.

degrees of degeneration. In one case, complete colliquation with
total hyalinization was observed in a fibroid mass of 3cm in
diameter, which had completely disappeared echographically.
      A different picture appeared in all other cases, in which
there were areas of hyalinization within the tissue with the
typical appearance of a leiomyoma (Fig 6). It is noteworth that
intense hyalinization was almost invariably observed around blood
vessels.

CONCLUSIONS

The present investigation shows that GnRH analogues produce a
substantial reduction in the volume of the uterus containing

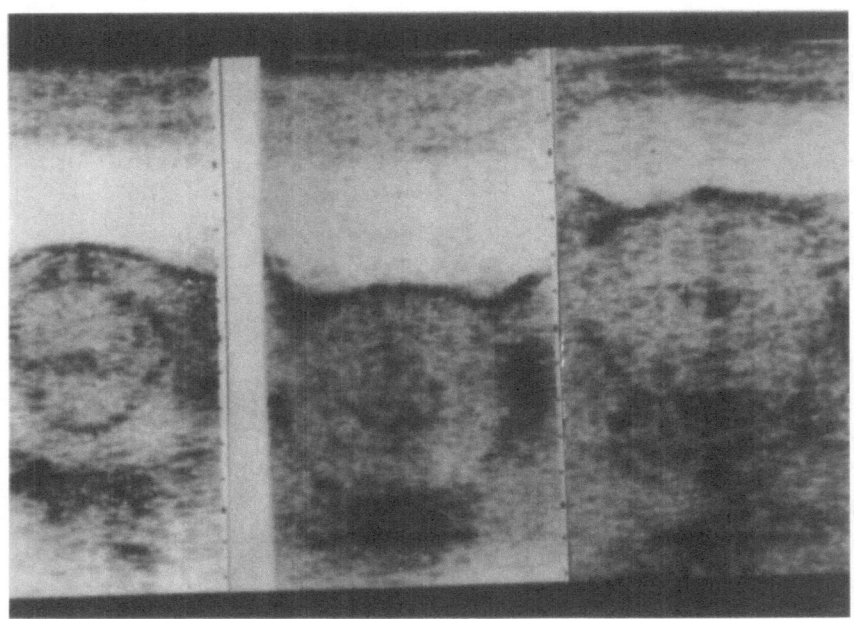

FIGURE 4   Ultrasound sequence demonstrating disappearance of a
myoma as therapy progresses.

leiomyomata. In the case of large uteri this may be due to the
reduction of leiomyomas. This is not the case for smaller uteri
where the reduction must be attributed to a decrease in size of
the organ itself.

In the present series the reduction in volume of fibroid
masses reached an average of 60%. This result is similar to that
observed in previous studies [10-15]. In contrast to other
reports [10, 11, 14], re-growth of the tumors did not occur in all
of the cases in the present study following discontinuation of
GnRH analogue therapy. In addition, the sequential use of MPA
stabilized fibroids at the size they reached at the end of
buserelin treatment, even when the progestogen was given at the
dose of only 25mg per day.

The administration of a GnRH agonist is invariably associated
with menopausal symptomatology [20, 21]. However, when the
frequency of various symptoms was compared in subjects treated

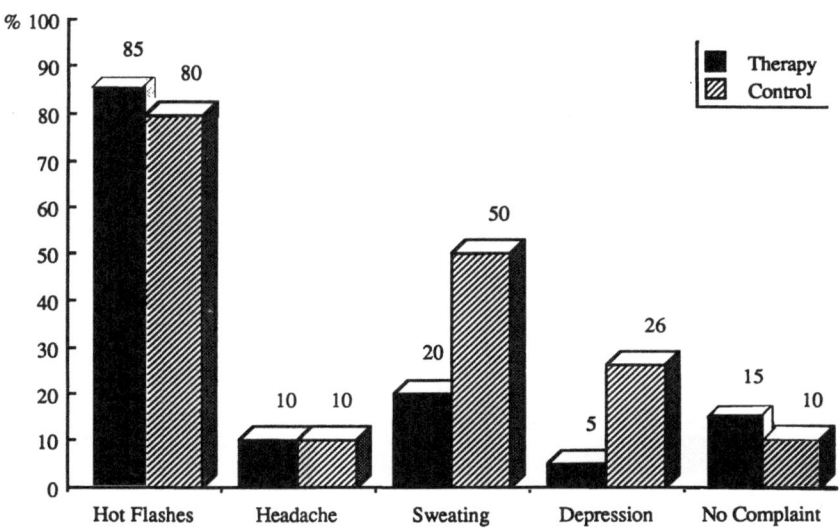

FIGURE 5   Incidence of side effects attributed to
     hypoestrogenism. The 45 cases treated with buserelin were
     compared with 50 healthy early menopausal women.

with buserelin and in healthy early menopausal women, there was a
significantly lower incidence of depression and sweating in the
first group.
     It is conceivable that treated women experienced less
depression because they had high motivation and knew that the
condition was transient. This would confirm the hypothesis that
depression is not directly correlated to hypoestrogenism [22].
There is little, if any, information in the literature concerning
histological changes due to GnRH agonist therapy. In the five
subjects undergoing surgery at the end of six months, various
degrees of hyalinization were observed in the fibroid masses,

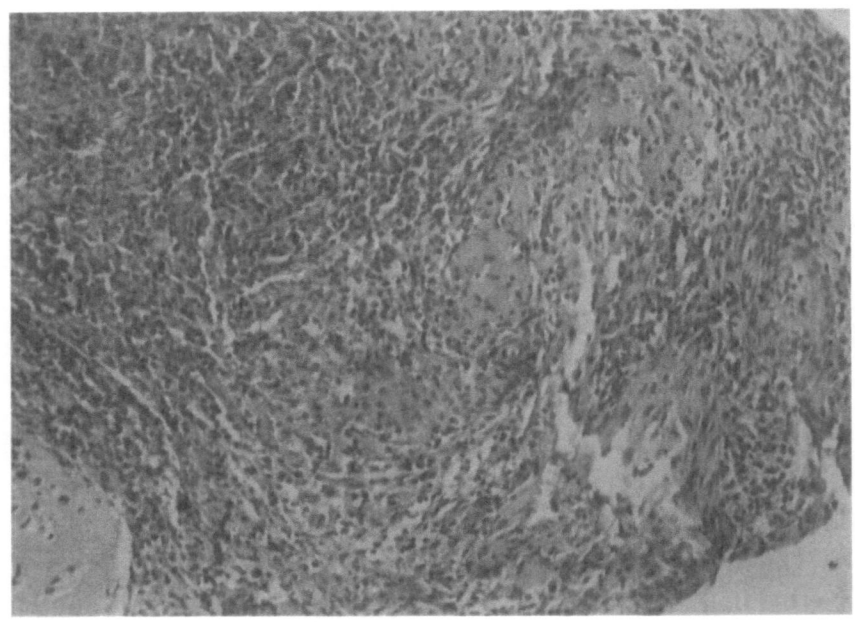

FIGURE 6 Histological appearance of leiomyoma following six
months of buserelin therapy. Areas of hyalinization appear
within the myomatous tissue which shows a lymphocytic
infiltration.

ranging from small areas within seemingly regular myomatous
tissue, to complete destruction of the tumour. This differing
responsivity may explain why only a certain percentage of the
tumours re-grow after stopping medication. Hyalinization was
invariably present in the perivascular tissue, suggesting that
decreased blood supply to the fibroid may play a role in the
regression.

No patient treated sequentially with buserelin and MPA has
required surgery and therefore no information is available on
histological changes induced by the progestogen.

REFERENCES

1. John, AH and Martin, R (1949). Growth of leiomyomata with estrogen-progesterone therapy. J Reprod Med, 6, 49
2. Goodman, AL (1946). Progesterone therapy in uterine fibroma. J Clin Endocrinol Metab, 9, 402
3. Segaloff, A, Weed, JC, Sternberg, WH and Parson, D (1949). The progesterone therapy of human uterine leiomyomas. J Clin Endocrinol Metab, 9, 1273
4. Goldzieher, JW, Maqueo, M, Ricaud, L, Aquilar, JH and Canales, E (1966). Induction of degenerative changes in uterine myomas by high dose progestin therapy. Am J Obstet Gynecol, 96, 1078
5. Hsueh, AJW, Peck, EJ and Clark, JH (1975). Progesterone antagonism of the oestrogen receptor and oestrogen induced uterine growth. Nature, 254, 337
6. Anderson, JN, Peck, EJ and Clark, JH (1975). Estrogen-induced uterine responses and growth: Relationship to receptors-estrogen binding by uterine nuclei. Endocrinology, 96, 160
7. Pukka, MJ, Kontula, KK, Kauppila, AJI, Janne, OA and Vihko, RK (1976). Estrogen receptor in human myoma tissue. Mol Cell Endocrinol, 6, 35
8. Soules, MR and McCarty, KS, Jr (1982). Leiomyomas: steroid receptor content. Variation within normal menstrual cycles. Am J Obstet Gynecol, 143, 6
9. Filicori, M, Hall, DA, Loughlin, JS, Rivier, J, Vale, W and Crowley, W, Jr. (1983). A conservative approach to the management of uterine leiomyoma: pituitary desensitization by a luteinizing hormone-releasing hormone analogue. Am J Obstet Gynecol, 147, 726
10. Healy, DL, Lawson, SR, Abbott, M, Baird, DT and Fraser, HM (1986). Toward removing uterine fibroids without surgery: subcutaneous infusion of a luteinizing hormone-releasing hormone agonist commencing in the luteal phase. J Clin Endocrinol Metab, 63, 619
11. Letterie, GS, Coddington, CC, Collins, RL, Shaker, TH, Anderson, R, Loriaux, DH and Winkel, CA (1986). Efficacy of Gn-RH analog (Gn-RH-a) in the treatment of uterine myomata: Long-term follow-up. Fertil Steril, 46, 3
12. Matta, W, Shaw, RV and Nye, M (1986). Studies of effect of a luteinizing hormone-releasing hormone (LHRH) agonist (buserelin) in patients with uterine leiomyomata. Brit J Obstet Gynecol, 93, 1194
13. Perl, V, Marquez, J, Schally, AV and Schally, AM (1987). Treatment of leiomyoma uteri with D-Trp6-luteinizing hormone-releasing hormone. Fertil Steril, 48, 383
14. Maheux, R, Lemay, A and Merat P (1987). Use of intranasal luteinizing hormone-releazing hormone agonist in uterine leiomyomas. Fertil Steril, 47, 229

15.   De Cecco, L, Costantini, S, Valenzano, M, Anserini, P, Orsi, F, Rissone, R and Venturini, PL (1987). Uso di un analogo agonista dell'LH-RH (buserelin) nella terapia dei fibromiomi uterini. In: Genazzani, AR, Volpe, A and Facchinetti, F (eds.) "Atti Seminario Invernale di Aggiornamento in Ginecologia e Ostetricia". vol.1, p.519. (Rome: CIC Edizioni Internazionali)
16.   Benagiano, G, Morini, A, Abbondante, G, Isidori, C and Latorre, PC (1987). Terapia medica del fibroleiomioma uterino. Risultati preliminari di uno studio comparitivo con danazolo, buserelin e medrossiprogesterone acetato. In: Genazzani, AR, Volpe, A and Facchinetti, F (eds.) "Atti Seminario Invernale di Aggiornamento in Ginecologia e Ostetricia". vol.2, p.9. (Rome: CIC Edizioni Internazionali)
17.   Morini, A, Primiero, FM, Napolitano, C, Latorre, PC, Aleandri, V and Benagiano, G (1987). Terapia medica sequenziale del fibromioma uterino con buserelin e progestinici. In: Fioretti, P and Melis, GB (eds.) "Atti 1° Congresso Nazionale di Scienze Ginecologiche ed Ostetriche" vol.1, p.189. (Rome: CIC Edizioni Internazionali)
18.   Primiero, FM, Morini, A, Abbondante, G, Caruso, G, Piccinno, F and Benagiano, G (1987). Terapia medica sequensiale del fibromioma uterino con danazolo e progestinici. In: Fioretti, P and Melis, GB (eds.) "Atti 1° Congresso Nazionale di Scienze Ginecologiche ed Ostetriche". vol.2 p.879. (Rome: CIC Edizioni Internazionali)
19.   Abbondante, G, Isidori, C, Latorre, PC, Marziani, R, Piccinno, F and Morini, A (1987). Aspetti ecografici della fibromatosi uterina e dell'endometrio in corso di terapia medica. In: Genazzani, AR, Volpe, A and Facchinetti F (eds.) "Atti Seminario Invernale di Aggiornamento in Ginecologia ed Ostetricia". vol.2, p.439. (Rome: CIC Edizioni Internazionali)
20.   Casper, RF, Yen SSC and Wilkes, MM (1981). Menopausal flushes: effect of pituitary gonadotropin desensitization by a potent luteinizing hormone-releasing factor agonist. J Clin Endocrinol Metab, 53, 1056
21.   De Fazio, HN, Meldrum, DR, Laufer, L, Vale, W, Rivier, J, Lu, KH and Judd, HL (1983). Induction of hot flushes in premenopausal women treated with a long-acting GnRH agonist. J Clin Endocrinol Metab, 56, 445
22.   Speroff, L, Glass, R, Case, N (1983). Clinical Gynecologic Endocrinology and Infertility. 3rd edition. (London:Williams & Wilkins)

7

COMBINED ENDOSCOPICAL AND ENDOCRINOLOGICAL TREATMENT OF UTERINE FIBROIDS

J.C. HUBER

1st Department of Gynecology and Obstetrics, A-1090 Vienna, Austria

INTRODUCTION

The preferred treatment for myoma uteri is total hysterectomy. Only in the case of desired fertility is the conservative management in form of a myomectomy commonly accepted.

We report on seven patients with uterine fibroids; three women were sterility patients and in four cases no more pregnancy was desired, there was only the serious intention to keep the uterus.

In sterility patients conservative surgery is widely used. Before laparotomy, we prefer laparoscopy for two reasons: Firstly, a more accurate diagnosis is possible and saves the time for a sometimes necessary consultation with surgeons or urologists. Secondly, the postsurgical formation of adhesions is reduced by endoscopic surgery, avoiding laparotomy.

In non sterility patients, two aspects for a conservative procedure should be considered: we have to respect the intention of some women to save their uterus and we have to keep in mind the reduced ovarian vascularisation and blood supply after hysterectomy. More than fifty percent of the arterial blood for ovarian nutrition emerges from the uterine vessels, going from the uterine artery over the mesosalpinx to the ovary. In the case of hysterectomy, this part of the ovarian vasculature is blocked and a consecutive ovarian insufficiency syndrome is observed. The so called "posthysterectomy syndrome" is similar to the climacterium praecox. Elevated gonadotropins and hot flushes are noted within one year in 20% of hysterectomized patients.

PRESENT STUDIES

Cytological screening of the cervix is obligatory, also the combined cytological and histological evaluation of the endometrium. We use therefore an instrument which is similar to an intrauterine device: in cases of cystic or atypic endometrial hyperplasia, hysterectomy is recommended. Another precaution is pretherapeutic screening for an early osteoporosis by single photon absorptiometry. A gamma ray source is placed on one side of the bone and a scintillation detector on the other. In high bone mineral losers, the GnRH analog treatment is not carried out at the moment.

Histological examination of the fibroids immediately after removal is also routine. This is an important advantage of our combined surgical and endocrinological treatment and allows us to register the cases of sarcomas.

The disadvantage of conservative myomectomy is a recurrence rate between ten and twenty-five percent. Despite myomectomy, the removal of all hypertrophic tissue is not practical. Therefore, postsurgical treatment with GnRH analogs is indicated to reduce the hypertrophic myoblasts and therefore also the recurrence of the fibroids.

The technique of our procedure has two aspects: the endoscopical enucleation followed by endocrinological treatment with GnRH analogs. The elimination of myoma pendulans by laparoscopy is easy: the so called Roeder loop is introduced intraabdominally through a 5 mm trochar sheath, closed, and the myoma cut down by endoscopical scissors. The removal of an intramyometrically localized fibroid is technically more difficult: normally we instill vasopressin round the myoma. This allows enucleation after the incision of the serosa without major bleeding.

The wound bed can be coagulated by bipolar hyperthermia or by laser. We use a Neodymiac laser which is introduced intraabdominally by a special applicator, which also allows the evacuation of the laser induced smoke. The hemostatic effect of fibrin can also be used in this surgical step; applied by endoscopical forceps, it covers the wound bed and replaces the serosa.

A real difficulty in endoscopical myomectomy is the elimination of isolated fibroids through the abdominal wall. Endocrinological treatment with the GnRH analog depot (decapeptyl) starts immediately after the surgical intervention. On the day after the laparoscopy, the first intramuscular injection is performed following by one injection per month over a period of half a year.

RESULTS

No signs of premature osteoporosis could be registered in the seven cases so treated. Histological examination of the endometrium excluded hyperplasia (Table 1).

Following the GnRH analog depot, every patient complained of hot flushes which started between one and three weeks after the injection. In 5 patients these symptoms were tolerable, in the others the analogs treatment was discontinued after 3 months.

Before laparoscopy and decapeptyl treatment, an intravaginal ultrasound examination of the uterine size and a documentation of the myomas were obligatory. Three months after the operation and after starting with decapeptyl a

Table 1. Characteristics of patients

Patients	Age	Position of Fibroids	Size of Fibroids	Continuance of Treatment	Hot Flushes
L.N.	35	subserosal	4 cm	6 months	+
L.K.	37	endometrial	4 cm	6 months	+
H.H.	38	subserosal	6 cm	3 months	+++
B.J.	32	subserosal	6 cm	4 months	+
F.N.	32	endometrial	3 cm	4 months	+
CH.R.	38	subserosal	3 cm	4 months	+
B.G.	38	subserosal + endometrial	4 cm 3 cm	4 months	+

control examination was carried out. The total uterine length was decreased on average between 0.5 cm and 1.5 cm compared to pretreatment. New myomas were not observed.

Table 2. Uterine dimensions before and after treatment

Patients	Before Treatment	After 3 Months
L.N.	9.5 cm	9 cm
L.K.	9 cm	8.5 cm
H.H.	9 cm	8.5 cm
B.J.	8.5 cm	8 cm
F.N.	10 cm	8.5 cm
CH.R.	9 cm	8.5 cm
B.G.	8.5 cm	8 cm

CONCLUSIONS

Decapeptyl has an additional growth reducing effect on the myometrium in addition to that achieved by surgery. The therapeutic effect is very high and there is no immediate recurrence.

8
NOVEL APPROACHES TO THE TREATMENT OF ADVANCED PROSTATE CANCER

A. MANNI, R. SANTEN, A. BOUCHER, A. LIPTON, H. HARVEY, M. SIMMONDS, D. WHITE-HERSHEY, M. BARTHOLOMEW, R. CAPLAN, R. GORDON, T. ROHNER, J. DRAGO, J. WETTLAUFER
and **L. GLODE**
Department of Medicine/Endocrinology,
The Milton S. Hershey Medical Center, The Pennsylvania State University,
PO Box 850, Hershey, PA 17033, USA

INTRODUCTION

Carcinoma of the prostate is the most common malignancy affecting men over the age of 55 and is the third leading cause of cancer death in this age group [1]. Unfortunately, more than half of the patients with prostatic carcinoma present with metastases (Stage D) at the time of diagnosis and have a mean survival of less than 2 years [2, 3]. The standard initial therapy of metastatic prostate cancer consists of castration either by surgical [4] or medical means with estrogens or, more recently, LHRH agonists [5]. The enthusiasm for this therapeutic approach is derived from the large fraction of patients (usually in excess of 80%) who experience both objective and subjective improvement. Unfortunately, however, the duration of response to castration is only, on average, 12-16 months [5, 6] and disease progression is associated with a 6 month survival of only 50% [2, 7]. Following relapse from the initial endocrine therapy, secondary hormonal treatment including antiandrogens, aminoglutethimide, surgical andrenalectomy and hypophysectomy induces objective tumor regression in only approximately 20% of the patients [8, 9]. A similarly low response rate has also been observed under these conditions with the use of cytotoxic chemotherapy [10]. Consequently, improved treatment strategies in this malignancy are urgently needed. In this review we will discuss novel approaches to the treatment of prostate cancer which may lead to an improved clinical outcome. The role of androgen priming as a potential means to improve response to cytotoxic chemotherapy as well as the potential merit of early combined endocrine therapy and chemotherapy will be reviewed. Finally, we will briefly discuss the potential usefulness in prostate cancer therapy of somatostatin analogs, a recently introduced class of compounds with possible antitumor action.

ANDROGEN PRIMING AND RESPONSE TO CYTOTOXIC CHEMOTHERAPY

Rationale

Prostate cancer cells may be subdivided into androgen-dependent and androgen-sensitive subpopulations. The dependent cohort requires androgens for cell viability and undergoes cell death upon androgen depletion. Androgen-sensitive cells, on the other hand, remain viable upon hormone depletion but revert either to G_0 or to a much slower proliferating state. With re-exposure to androgens these cells resume active proliferation. The surviving androgen-sensitive cells may undergo adaptation with subsequent resumption of growth and may thus be responsible for tumor progression following response to the initial endocrine therapy. The mechanism for the adaptation of the androgen-sensitive cells to survive in an androgen-deprived milieu are unknown but could reflect frequent rearrangements of chromosomal DNA, a phenomenon recently recognized in tumor tissue [11]. The development of androgen-independent growth occurring after androgen deprivation has recently been studied in a model system. The androgen-dependent Shionogi mouse mammary tumor cell line retains the ability to grow more rapidly in the presence of androgen provided that it is continuously exposed to androgen. In marked contrast, within weeks of androgen deprivation, these cells become androgen-independent and regrow rapidly [12, 13]. This escape from androgen sensitivity does not result from loss of androgen receptors but is associated with loss of a series of receptor-mediated functions. The proliferation rate of these cells increases as the process of hormone independency develops and the degree of in vitro contact inhibition diminishes.

Based upon these concepts it would then be critical to eliminate androgen-sensitive cells in patients to prevent their later regrowth. Since these cells are quiescent following androgen depletion they may be relatively insensitive to the action of cytotoxic therapy which is more effective against rapidly dividing cells [14]. It may, however, be possible to take advantage of the androgen sensitivity of these cells by transiently stimulating their growth with exogenous androgen administration in order to enhance their sensitivity to cytotoxic chemotherapy.

Basic Studies and Pilot Clinical Trials Testing the Effect of Androgen Priming

A variety of experimental data is available to support the ability of androgens to stimulate and synchronize proliferation of normal and neoplastic prostatic tissue [15-20]. Preliminary experimental data also suggests that the cytotoxic effect of chemotherapy can be potentiated if administered during hormone-induced cell synchronization and recruitment. Sufrin et al [21] observed that adriamycin administration to castrated rats at the peak of testosterone-stimulated prostatic DNA synthesis was able to produce a greater destruction of normal prostatic tissue than under control conditions. Grossman et al [22] tested the concept of androgen priming in the treatment of the Dunning R-3227G androgen-dependent prostate tumor. These investigators observed that the ability of methotrexate to inhibit tumor growth was significantly potentiated by transient androgen priming.

More than 20 years ago several investigators attempted to enhance the antitumor effect of 32P by prior transient androgen administration in men with advanced prostate cancer [23-25]. The androgen priming was designed to increase the uptake of the isotope into the tumor and thereby increase tumor cell kill. Although the regimen was effective in reducing bone pain the exact role of androgen priming was not clear. Treatment strategies of hormonal stimulation plus chemotherapy have recently been applied to the treatment of advanced prostate cancer in humans. Kedia et al [26] reported an 85% response rate (tumor regression + stabilization) in 30 men with stage D prostate cancer given testosterone propionate for 3 days before administration of cyclophosphamide, cisplatinum and 5-fluorouracil. Such a high response rate suggested that the antitumor effect of chemotherapy may have been enhanced by androgen priming. In contrast, Suarez et al [27] demonstrated only a 43% objective rate of regression or stabilization in 21 men treated with fluoxymesterone followed by cyclophosphamide and methotrexate. The authors concluded that these therapeutic results were not superior to those reported with the use of cytotoxic drugs alone. Since, however, neither study included a control group, no firm conclusion could be drawn on the potential merit of this novel therapeutic approach.

Prospective Randomized Clinical Trials

Over the last 6 years we have conducted a randomized clinical trial in patients with Stage D-2 prostate cancer refractory to orchiectomy to test whether androgen priming potentiates the effect of cytotoxic chemotherapy. Interim analyses of the data have been published [28-30]. A total of 85 patients have been entered into the study of whom 41 have been randomized to the stimulation and 44 to the control arm. Although the patients were not stratified prior to randomization both groups were comparable with regard to several characteristics including age, performance status, baseline hematocrit, time from castration, extent of metastatic involvement, proportion of patients with elevated acid phosphatase levels and previous systemic therapy. The median duration of follow-up is 43 months (range: 7-71 months). Only 10% of the patients are still living. At the time of entry into the study all patients had evidence of progressive and evaluable disease following orchiectomy. In addition, half of the patients had also received estrogen therapy while no one had received previous systemic cytotoxic chemotherapy.

All patients were chronically treated with aminoglutethimide (1gm daily) and hydrocortisone (40mg daily) to lower adrenal androgen secretion. All patients were also treated with intravenous cyclic chemotherapy every 3 weeks which consisted initially of 500mg/M^2 cyclophosphamide, 500mg/M^2 5-fluorouracil and 50mg/M^2 adriamycin. After a maximum cumulative dose of 400mg/M^2 of adriamycin the chemotherapy was changed to 200mg/M^2 methotrexate followed 1 hour later by 600mg/M^2 5-fluorouracil and 24 h later by 10mg/M^2 citrovorum factor rescue 4 times daily for a total of 6 doses. This later combination chemotherapy was given every 4 weeks. Patients who were randomized to the stimulation arm received the synthetic androgen fluoxymesterone (5mg orally twice a day) for 3 days before and on the day of chemotherapy administration. The treatment was continued until there was evidence of progressive disease. The criteria of response employed were those of the National Prostatic Cancer Project [31] with the exception that a 50% decrease rather than a normalization of the acid phosphatase was required to classify a patient as an objective responder. This modification was indroduced because a fraction of patients showed clear evidence of objective remission on x-rays and/or scans despite the failure of the serum acid phosphatase to normalize.

Response rate was slightly but not significantly higher in the control than in the stimulation arm (Table 1). The 95% confidence interval for the difference in response rate is between 36% in favor of control and 6% in favor of stimulation. Of the patients who benefited from the treatment, approximately half obtained actual objective tumor regression while the other half only obtained disease stabilization. When our analysis was restricted to only evaluable patients a similar high response rate was observed in the two arms of the protocol (79% and 73% for the stimulation and control arm, respectively). A larger proportion of unevaluable patients were noted in the stimulation compared to the control arm (42% vs. 16%) which was due, at least in part, to fluoxymesterone toxicity resulting in early discontinuation of the protocol treatment. Median duration of objective remission and disease stabilization was not statistically significant between the control and the stimulation arms. When patients with objective remission and disease stabilization are considered together the median duration of response was 10 months for the control group and 9 months for the stimulation arm (p=.1725, Mantel-Cox).

Median survival was significantly longer in the control compared to the stimulation arm (15 months vs. 10 months, p=.0047, Mantex-Cox). When the patients in both groups are considered together the median duration of survival was 24 months for patients with objective remissions, 13 months for those with stable disease, 7 months for failures and 6 months for unevaluable patients.

Toxicity from the protocol treatment was primarily associated with androgen priming. Three patients developed reversible neurological compromise during the first cycle of androgen priming. In two, this was due to spinal cord compression while, in the third, the etiology of the neurological deficit remained undetermined. Most patients

Table I. Response rate and duration in the two arms of the protocol

	Stimulation Arm (N=41)			Control Arm (N=44)		
	No. of Patients	%	Median Duration of Response (Months)	No. of Patients	%	Median Duration of Response (Months)
Remissions	10	24	10	13	29	18
		46			61	
Stable disease	9	22	3	14	32	6
Failures	5	12	--	10	23	--
Unevaluable[a]	17	42	--	7	16	--

[a]Patients were considered to be unevaluable if they had not received at least 2 cycles of hormone priming plus chemotherapy or chemotherapy alone.

experienced exacerbation of bone pain during androgen priming which necessitated discontinuation of the treatment in 2. Of the 17 unevaluable patients in the stimulation arm, early discontinuation of treatment was directly related to androgen priming toxicity in 5. It is worth noting, however, that the bone pain flare decreased in most patients and disappeared completely in a few after several cycles of therapy. This finding indicates that, once the tumor burden has been reduced by cytotoxic drugs, androgen priming no longer had major deleterious clinical consequences. No major toxicity was observed with aminoglutethimide plus hydrocortisone and cytotoxic chemotherapy except for two cases of adriamycin-induced congestive heart failure.

We believe that the largely negative data of our randomized trial with regard to the role of androgen priming can probably best be explained by the late stage of disease when the treatment was instituted. It is likely that the high tumor burden present in our patients may have placed them at a particlarly high risk of toxicity from androgen priming. Furthermore, patients with a large tumor burden may be intrinsically more resistant to cytotoxic drugs and thus may be less manipulable in this regard by hormonal means. Consequently, we feel that this treatment strategy should probably be tested earlier in the course of the disease before or simultaneously with the initial castration when a smaller tumor burden is present and when, perhaps, a larger fraction of tumor cells are hormone-responsive.

POTENTIAL IMPORTANCE OF EARLY COMBINED HORMONAL THERAPY AND CHEMOTHERAPY IN THE TREATMENT OF PROSTATE CANCER

The conventional approach to the treatment of prostate cancer is to reserve cytotoxic chemotherapy to the later stages of the disease at the time of progression following hormonal therapy. As mentioned above, under these conditions, chemotherapy only meets with limited success. A possible reason for the relative ineffectiveness of cytotoxic drugs in patients with refractory Stage D prostate cancer is the late stage of disease when the treatment is administered. Theoretical considerations support the hypothesis that cancers at a late stage with a large tumor burden may be less likely to respond to therapy. One consideration involves the somatic mutation theory of carcinogenesis which has found support from studies on the development of retinoblastoma [32] and Wilm's tumors [33]. According to this theory, cancer development occurs following errors resulting in somatic mutation of two good gene copies or of only a single gene copy if a bad gene copy has been inherited. Tumor progression may then be associated with increasing numbers of subsequent errors occurring in a cascade fashion with time and yielding at the end an aggressive tumor, poorly responsive to therapy. This idea parallels the thinking of Orgel [34] who used an error cascade theory to explain aging. The degree of aggressiveness should then correlate with the number of population doublings undergone since the initiating event. If so, early tumors will be qualitatively different (i.e., less aggressive and more amenable to therapy) from late tumors.

An additional theoretical consideration involves the possibility of phenotypic lag in expressing a given characteristic such as possible sensitivity to chemotherapy. If a tumor becomes detectable at 10^9 cells and kills the host at 10^{12} there are only 10 population doublings between diagnosis and patient's death. Since phenotypic lag can expand up to 7 generations, as shown for the expression of 6 thioguanine resistance [35], one must intervene with effective chemotherapy very early in order to have a significant impact on the patient's survival.

Recent experimental evidence provides support for early theraputic intervention in the treatment of prostate cancer. In a series of detailed experiments, Isaacs [36] evaluated the role of timing of androgen ablation therapy and/or chemotherapy in the treatment of prostatic cancer using, as a model, the transplant- able, well-differentiated, androgen-sensitive Dunning R-3327H rat prostatic adenocarcinoma. This investigator first evaluated the effect of castration performed at different times after tumor inoculation on tumor growth and animal survival. He found that actual tumor regression occurred only in the animals that were castrated early whereas in those castrated later only a decrease in the rate in tumor growth was observed. More importantly, he found a highly significant negative correlation between average survival after tumor inoculation and time of castration. Similarly, administration of cytoxan was able to prolong animal survival only when administered early. When cytoxan treatment was begun late it actually significantly decreased overall host survival compared to the control untreated group. The best therapeutic results were obtained when both treatments were given simultaneously and early. In contrast, sequential therapy involving early castration followed by delayed cytoxan administration, or the reverse sequence, had no effect on survival compared to untreated animals. Combined therapy instituted late was actually associated with a significantly shorter survival.

Some support for early initiation of combined hormonal therapy and chemotherapy in patients with stage D prostate cancer has also been provided by a pilot clinical trial [37] Combination of endocrine and chemotherapy initiated soon after diagnosis of stage D prostate cancer was associated with a cumulative survival rate during 3-1/2 years of 76.5%. These survival data seem to compare favorably to results obtained with castration alone.

SOMATOSTATIN ANALOGUES AS POTENTIALLY USEFUL AGENTS IN THE TREATMENT OF ADVANCED PROSTATE CANCER

Somatostatin analogues are a new class of compounds with potentially broad application in the treatment of human tumors. They have been demonstrated to be effective in the treatment of refractory acromegaly [38-40], as well as a variety of other endocrine tumors [41-44]. Some preliminary evidence suggests that these drugs may also be useful in the treatment of other malignancies such as breast [45] and prostate cancer [46]. The rationale for the potential mechanisms of action of the somatostatin analogues in the treatment of prostate cancer involves the following considerations: Their antitumor action could be mediated, in part, through suppression of growth hormone and, at times, prolactin secretion. Prolactin has, in fact, been postulated to be involved as a co-factor in prostatic cancer growth [47-51]. The beneficial effect of suppression of growth hormone secretion may be due to the lowering of circulating levels of important growth factors, such as IGF-1, which are under growth hormone control. Somatostatin analogues may also directly interfere with autocrine/ paracrine mechanisms affecting neoplastic proliferation. Somatostatin has been found to inhibit the cell replication induced by epidermal growth factor (EGF) [52]. In a human pacreatic cancer cell line somatostatin has been shown to reverse the stimulatory effect of GEF on the phosphorylation of the tyrosine kinase portion of the EGF receptor [53]. Thus, somatostatin analogues may directly inhibit the action of endogenous growth factors, such as EFG, by interference with signal transmission.

Recently, Schally and Redding tested the usefulness of somatostatin analogues as adjuncts to LHRH agonists in the treatment of the Dunning R-3327H rat prostate cancer model

73

[46]. The analogues significantly retarded tumor growth when administered alone and also potentiated the antitumor effect of the LHRH agonists. These encouraging preliminary results provide a rationale for testing these compounds, perhaps in conjunction with standard endocrine therapy in the treatment of prostate cancer in humans.

REFERENCES

1.   Silverberg, E (1985). Cancer statistics. Cancer, 35, 19
2.   Klein, LA (1979). Medical progress: prostatic carcinoma. New Engl J Med, 300, 824
3.   Schoones, R, Palma, LD, Gaeta, JF, Moore, RH and Murphy, GP (1972). Prostatic carcinoma treated at categorical center: Clinical and pathological observations. NY State J. Med, 72, 1021
4.   Huggins, C, Stevens, Jr, RE and Hodges, CV (1941). Studies on prostatic cancer. II. The effects of castration on advanced carcinoma of the prostate gland. Arch Surg, 43, 209
5.   The Leuprolide Study Group (1984). Leuprolide versus diethylstilbestrol for metastatic prostate cancer. New Engl J Med, 311, 1281
6.   Smith, JA Jr, (1984). Androgen suppression by a gonadotropin releasing hormone analogue in patients with metastatic carcinoma of the prostate. J Urol, 131, 1110
7.   Johnson, DE, Scott, WW, Gibbons, RP, Prout, GR, Smidt, JD, Chu, TM, Gaeta, J, Saroff, J and Murphy, GP (1977). National randomized study of chemotherapeutic agents in advanced prostatic carcinoma: a progress report. Cancer Treat Rep, 61, 317
8.   Resnick, MI and Grayhack, JT (1975). Treatment of stage IV carcinoma of the prostate. Urol Clin N Amer, 2, 141
9.   Drago, JR, Santen, RJ, Lipton, A, Worgul, TJ, Harvey, HA, Boucher, A, Manni, A and Rohner, TJ (1984). Clinical effect of aminogluethimide, medical adrenalectomy, in treatment of 43 patients with advanced prostatic carcinoma. Cancer, 53, 1447
10.   Torti, FM and Carter, SK (1980). The chemotherapy of prostatic adenocarcinoma. Ann Int Med, 92, 681
11.   Cairns, J (1981). The origin of human cancers. Nature, 289, 353
12.   Darbre, P and King, RJB (1987). Progression to steroid autonomy in S115 mouse mammary tumor cells: Role of DNA methylation. J Cell Biol, 99, 1410
13.   Darbre, P and King, RJB (1987). Differential effects of steroid hormones on parameters of cell growth. Cancer Res 47, 2937
14.   Sulkes, A, Livingston, RB and Murphy, WK (1979). Tritiated thymidine labelling index and response in human breast cancer. J Natl Cancer Inst, 62, 513
15.   Tuohimaa, P and Niemi, M (1968). The effect of testosterone on cell renewal and mitotic cycles in sex accessory glands of castrated mice. Acta Endocrinol, 58, 696

16.   Sufrin, G and Coffey, DS (1973). A new model for studying the effect of drugs on prostatic growth. I. Antiandrogens and DNA synthesis. Invest Urol, 11, 45
17.   Lesser, B and Bruchovsky, N (1973). The effects of testosterone, 5α-dihydrotestosterone and adenosine 3',5'-monophosphate on cell proliferation and differentiation in rat prostate. Biochem Biophys Acta, 308, 426
18.   Sufrin, G and Coffey, DS (1975). Differences in the mechanism of action of medrogestone and cyproterone acetate. Invest Urol, 13, 1
19.   McMahon, MJ, Butler, AVJ and Thomas, GH (1972). Morphological responses of prostatic carcinoma to testosterone in organ culture. Brit J Cancer, 26, 388
20.   English, HF, Kloszewski, ED, Valentine, E and Santen, RJ (1986). Proliferative response of the Dunning R-3327H experimental model of prostatic adenocarcinoma to conditions of androgen depletion and repletion. Cancer Res, 46, 839
21.   Sufrin, G, Heston, W, Llado, J and Coffey, D (1979). The role of cell proliferation on the response to chemotherapy in the rat prostate. Amer Urol Assoc, p. 205 (Abstr 433)
22.   Grossman, HB, Kleinert, EL, Lesser, ML, Herr, HW and Whitmore, Jr, WF (1981). Androgen stimulated chemotherapy in the Dunnning R-3327 prostatic adenocarcinoma. Urol Res, 9, 237
23.   Donati, RM, Ellis, H and Gallager, NI (1966). Testosterone potentiated 32P therapy in prostatic carcinoma. Cancer, 19, 1088
24.   Edland, RW (1974). Testosterone potentiated radiophos-phorous therapy of osseous metastases in prostate cancer. Am J Roentgenology, 120, 678
25.   Maxfield, JR, Maxfield, JGS and Maxfield, WS (1958). The use of radioactive phosphorous and testosterone in metastatic bone lesions from breast and prostate. S Med J, 51, 320
26.   Kedia KR, Kellermeyer, RW and Perskey, L (1981). Hormonal stimulation followed by multiagent chemotherapy in estrogen unresponsive prostatic adenocarcinoma. Proc Amer Urol Assoc, p. 191A
27.   Suarez, AJ, Lamm, DL, Radwin, HM, Sarosdy, M, Clark, G and Osborne, DK (1982). Androgen priming and cytotoxic chemotherapy in advanced prostatic cancer. Cancer Chemother Pharmacol, 18, 261
28.   Manni, A, Santen, RJ, Boucher, A, Harvey, H, Simmonds, M, White, D, Gordon, R, Rohner, T, Drago, J, Wettlaufer, J and Glode, LM (1985). Hormone stimulation and chemotherapy in advanced prostate cancer: Preliminary results of a prospective controlled clinical trial. Anticancer Res, 5, 161
29.   Manni, A, Santen, RJ, Boucher, AE, Lipton, A, Harvey, H, Simmonds, M, White-Hershey, D, Gordon, RA, Rohner, TJ, Drago, J, Wettlaufer, J and Glode, LM (1986). Hormone stimulation and chemotherapy in advanced prostate cancer: Interim analysis of an ongoing randomized trial. Anticancer Res, 6, 309
30.   Manni, A, Santen, RJ, Boucher, AE, Lipton, A, Harvey, H, Simmonds, M, White-Hershey, D, Gordon, RA, Rohner, TJ, Drago, J, Wettlaufer, J and Glode, LM (1986). Androgen priming and

response to chemotherapy in advanced prostatic cancer. J Urol, 136, 1242

31.   Murphy, GR and Slack, NH (1980). Response criteria for the prostate of the USA National Prostatic Cancer Project. The Prostate, 1, 375

32.   Yunis, JJ and Ramsey, N (1978). Retinoblastoma and subband deletion of chromosome 13. Am J Dis, 132, 161

33.   Weissman, BE, Saxon, PJ, Pasquale, SR, Jones, GR, Geiser, AG and Stanbridge, EJ (1987). Introduction of a normal human chromosome 11 into a Wilms' tumor cell line controls its tumorigenic expression. Science, 236, 175

34.   Orgel, LE (1963). The maintenance of accuracy of protein synthesis and its relevance to aging. Proc Natl Acad Sci USA, 49, 517

35.   Penman, BW and Thilly, WG (1976). Concentration-dependent mutation of diploid human lymphoblasts by methylnitrosoguanidine: The importance of phenotypic lag. Somat Cell Gen, 2, 325

36.   Isaacs, JT (1984). The timing of androgen ablation therapy and/or chemotherapy in the treatment of prostatic cancer. The Prostate, 5, 1

37.   Mukamel, E, Nissenkorn, I and Servadio, C (1980). Early combined hormonal and chemotherapy for metastatic carcinoma of the prostate. Urology, 16, 257

38.   Barkan, AL, Kelch,RP, Hopwood, NJ and Beitins, IZ (1988). Treatment of acromegaly with the long-acting somatostatin analog SMS 201-995. J Clin Endocrinol Metab, 66, 16

39.   Lamberts, SWJ, Uitterlinden, P and Del Pozo, E (1987). SMS 201-995 induces a continuous decline in circulating growth hormone and somatomedin-C levels during therapy of acromegalic patients for over two years. J Clin Endocrinol Metab, 65, 703

40.   Chiodini, PG, Cozzi, R, Dallabonzana, D, Oppizzi, G, Verde, G, Petroncini, M, Liuzzi, A and Del Pozo, E (1987). Medical treatment of acromegaly with SMS 201-995, a somatostatin analog: a comparison with bromocriptine. J Clin Endocrinol Metab, 64, 447

41.   Geehoed, GW, Bass, BL, Mertz, SL and Becker, KL (1986). Somatostatin analog: effects on hypergastrinemia and hypercalcitonemia. Surgery, 6, 962

42.   Santangelo, WC, O'Dorisio, TM, Kim, JG, Severino, G and Krejs, GJ (1985). Pancreatic cholera syndrome: Effect of a synthetic somatostatin analog on intestinal water and ion transport. Ann Int Med, 103, 363

43.   Altimari, AF, Bhoopalam, N, O'Dorisio, T, Lange, CL, Sandberg, L, and Prinz, RA (1986). Use of a somatostatin analog (SMS 201-995) in the glucagonoma syndrome. Surgery, 6, 989

44.   Boden, G, Ryan, IG, Eisenschmid, BL, Shelmet, JJ and Owen, OE (1986). Treatment of inoperable glucagonoma with the long-acting somatostatin analogue SMS 201-995. New Engl J Med, 314, 1686

45. Setyono-Han, B, Henkelman, MS, Foekens, JA and Klijn, JGM (1987). Direct inhibitory effect of somatostatin (analogues) on the growth of human breast cancer cells. Cancer Res, 74, 1566

46. Schally, AV and Redding, TW (1987). Somatostatin analogs as adjuncts to agonists of luteinizing hormone-releasing hormone in the treatment of experimental prostate cancer. Proc Natl Acad Sci USA, 84, 7275

47. Assimos, D. Smith, C, Lee, C and Grayhack, JT (1984). Action of prolactin in regressing prostate: Independent action mediated by androgen receptors. The Prostate, 5, 589

48. Holland, RM and Lee, C (1980). Effects of hyper-prolactinemia on the accessory steroidogenesis of the male rat. Biol Reprod, 22, 351

49. Coert, A, Nievelstein, H, Kloosterboer, HJ, Loonen, P and Van der Vries, J (1985). Effects of pituitary grafts on testosterone stimulated growth of rat prostate. The Prostate, 6, 269

50. Johnson, MP, Thompson, SA and Lubaroff, DM (1985). Differential effects of prolactin on rat dorsolateral prostate and R-3327 prostate tumor sublines. J Urol, 133, 1112

51. Muntzing, J, Kirdani, R, Murphy, GP and Sandberg, AA (1977). Hormonal control of zinc uptake and binding in the rat dorsolateral prostate. Invest Urol, 14, 492

52. Mascardo, RN and Sherline, P (1982). Somatostatin inhibits rapid intrasomal separation and cell proliferation induced by epidermal growth factor. Endocrinology, 111, 1394

53. Hierowski, MT, Leibow, C, Sapin, K and Schally, AV (1985). Stimulation by somatostatin of dephosphorylation of membrane proteins in pancreatic cancer MIA PaCA-2 cell line. FEBS Lett, 179, 252

9

MAXIMAL ANDROGEN BLOCKAGE IN PROSTATE CANCER: TODAY'S THERAPY OF CHOICE AND 5-YEAR CLINICAL EXPERIENCE

Fernand LABRIE, André DUPONT, Lionel CUSAN, Gilles MANHÈS, Yves LACOURCIÈRE, Gérard MONFETTE and Jean EMOND
Departments of Molecular Endocrinology, Medicine, Nuclear Medicine and Urology, Laval University Medical Center, Quebec G1V 4G2, Canada

INTRODUCTION

Prostate cancer is the second leading cause of death due to cancer in men [1]. In fact, this disease has reached the frequency of lung cancer and it was estimated that 96,000 new cases would be discovered in the United States in 1987 [1]. Among these patients, approximately 59% are at an advanced stage with bone metastases already present at the time of first diagnosis, thus making endocrine manipulations the only efficient therapy available.

Since the original observations of Huggins and his colleagues who demonstrated the role of testicular androgens in prostate cancer [2], all the successful approaches have involved various degrees of blockade of androgens [3]. Almost all procedures, however, were limited to the blockade of testicular androgens. The relatively recent information on the serious and frequently lethal cardiovascular complications of estrogens [4, 5] and estramustine phosphate [6] clearly indicates that today's choice for the blockade of testicular androgens is between orchiectomy and the extremely well tolerated LHRH agonists [3, 7, 8].

Man, however, unlike any other mammalian species, possesses adrenals which secrete large amount of precursor steroids which are converted into active androgens in the peripheral tissues, especially the normal prostate and prostate cancer [9]. In fact, following chemical or surgical castration, 30 to 50% of the most active natural androgen, namely dihydrotestosterone (DHT), remains in the prostatic cancer tissue [3, 10]. In order to take into account this new but already well documented information [10], a more complete blockade of androgens using a pure antiandrogen in association with chemical or surgical castration has been developed and has shown objective advantages compared with standard therapies limited to the blockade of testicular androgens [3, 10-13], with no significant side effect.

While the rationale supporting maximal androgen blockade for the optimal therapy of prostate cancer is well documented [3, 10, 14], it seems appropriate to summarize the clinical data obtained using this approach in prostate cancer patients at various stages of the disease and with various pretreatments.

ELIMINATION OF THE RISK OF DISEASE FLARE

It currently is well established that castration levels of serum androgens can be achieved by chronic administration of agonists of LHRH without side effects other than those related to hypoandrogenism, namely hot flashes and a decrease or loss of libido and sexual potency [7, 11, 15-19]. These exceptionally well tolerated peptides offer an alternative therapy devoid of the side effects of estrogens and free of the psychological limitations of orchiectomy. However, as observed in the first patient with prostatic cancer treated with an LHRH agonist [7], a limitation to the use of such agonists alone is the transient increase in serum testosterone (and dihydrotestosterone) resulting from increased secretion of LH induced by the LHRH agonist during the first 5-10 days of treatment with the now well-recognized risk of disease flare in a significant proportion of patients [20-23]. At later intervals complete pituitary desensitization occurs [23], thus leading to a decrease in serum testosterone and dihydrotestosterone concentrations to castration levels for as long as treatment continues [3, 7, 8, 11, 15-19, 24].

To block the harmful effect of the increase in serum androgens on cancer growth, we have administered the antiandrogen Flutamide, a blocker of the androgen receptor [25, 26] in association with the LHRH agonist [D-Trp^6,Pro^{9}NHEt]LHRH to more than 1000 patients with advanced prostate cancer during the last 5 years with no sign or symptom of disease flare in any patient. Considering the wide use of LHRH agonists for the treatment of prostatic cancer, we performed simultaneous measurements of serum testosterone and prostatic acid phosphatase (PAP) in seventy patients with previously untreated advanced (with bone metastases) prostatic cancer during the first month of combination therapy with Flutamide and [D-Trp^6,Pro^{9}NHEt]LHRH. Careful clinical evaluation of pain, performance and other relevant symptoms and signs also was performed in order to detect any sign of disease flare. These data show that simultaneous treatment with the LHRH agonist and antiandrogen causes a rapid improvement of the disease with no sign or symptom of disease exacerbation in any patient. On the contrary, early clinical improvement was already observed in a significant proportion of patients during the first week of combined treatment.

Three days after the first daily injection of the LHRH agonist in patients simultaneously treated with the

80

antiandrogen, serum testosterone was 47% increased above pretreatment values (p ≤0.01). At 7 days, serum testosterone had decreased to 15% above conrol (N.S.) while at 12, 19 and 30 days, it was decreased to 50, 16 and 10% of control, respectively (p ≤0.01, part A of Figure 1).

Since the levels of serum PAP are a sensitive, precise and objective biological marker of androgen action in androgen-sensitive prostatic cancer tissue, it is of great interest to see in Fig. 1B that the serum PAP concentration is already decreased to 36% of pretreatment values on day 3 of combined treatment (p <0.01) are measured at the later time intervals (7, 13 and 30 days).

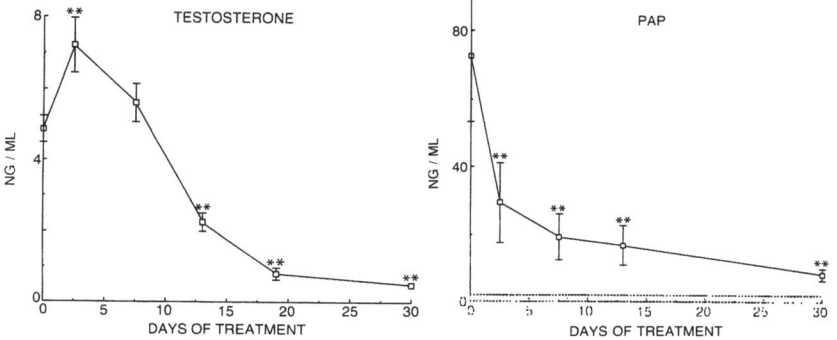

FIGURE 1   Serum response to daily subcutaneous administration of 500µg, (D-Trp[6], Pro[9]NHEt)LHRH ethylamide in association with oral flutamide (250mg, every 8 hours) begun 24 hours before first injection of LHRH agonist in 70 previously untreated patients with stage D2 prostate cancer. Bars represent standard error of mean. **, p<0.01, A, serum testosterone concentration. B, serum prostatic acid phosphatase (PAP) concentration.

In agreement with the rapid and marked decrease in serum PAP levels during the first days of treatment, there was no increase in pain or worsening of the performance status during the first weeks of treatment in any patient. On the contrary, pain was decreased appreciably in 7 patients within a week. After 2 weeks, pain had already disappeared in 7 patients and decreased in 20 other subjects. At one month, pain had disappeared in 18 (44%) of 41 patients who has this symptom at the start of treatment. Moreover, severe pain (grade 3+ or 4+) originally present in 10 patients, was no longer present in any patient. Moderate pain (2+) was present in only 4 patients aftr 1 month of treatment as compared to 26 who had grade (2+) was present in only 4 patients after 1 month of treatment compared with grade 2# (or more) pain before treatment.

Problems of performance were observed in 34 patients at the start of treatment, including 7 in bed for more than 50 per cent of the time and 2 in bed 100 per cent of the time. Performance became normal in 7 patients within 1 week of treatment and it became normal in 20 within 1 month. At 1 month, no patient remained bedridden for more than 50 per cent of the time and only 5 had to stay in bed for some time compared to 18 at the start of treatment, with 2 being completely bedridden.

The recent report of Waxman and associates should provide the final argument that the use of LHRH agonists alone for advanced prostatic cancer has an unacceptable risk of tumor flare or exacerbation of the signs and symptoms of cancer [22].

COMBINATION THERAPY IN PREVIOUSLY UNTREATED STAGE D2 PATIENTS

As mentioned above, a recently recognized characteristic of human prostate cancer is that man is unique among species in having a high secretion rate of adrenal steroids which are converted into potent androgens in the prostatic tissue itself. An endocrine finding of major importance in this field is the discovery that androgens of adrenal origin can play a role comparable to that of androgens of testicular origin in the growth of prostate cancer[3]. In addition to convincing biochemical evidence [27, 28], the unequivocal role of adrenal androgens in the growth of human prostate cancer is clearly demonstrated by the numerous studies showing a 30 to 60% objective response to hypophysectomy, aminoglutethimide or Flutamide in patients in relapse after orchiectomy or estrogen treatment [3, 29-34].

In order to achieve a more complete blockade of androgens, we have combined pure antiandrogen with castration (chemical with an LHRH agonist or orchiectomy) at the start of treatment of 199 patients presenting with clinical stage D2 prostate cancer without previous endocrine therapy.

The efficacy of the combination therapy was assessed by analysis of: 1 best objective response, measured according to the criteria of the US NPCP [36]; 2 duration of objective response, measured according to the same criteria and 3 survival (Fig. 2). Since the results obtained using the same objective criteria in many recent studies on the blockade of testicular androgens achieved by various approaches have yielded almost super-imposable results [21, 36, 37], thus indicating the reliability of the criteria used, we have compared the present results with those obtained in recent studies performed with comparable populations of patients who started treatment at the same stage of the disease.

As illustrated in Fig. 3, a positive objective response assessed according to the criteria of the US NPCP[35] has been obtained in 174 of 186 patients (93.5%), thus leaving only 12 patients (6.5%) with no response at the start of the

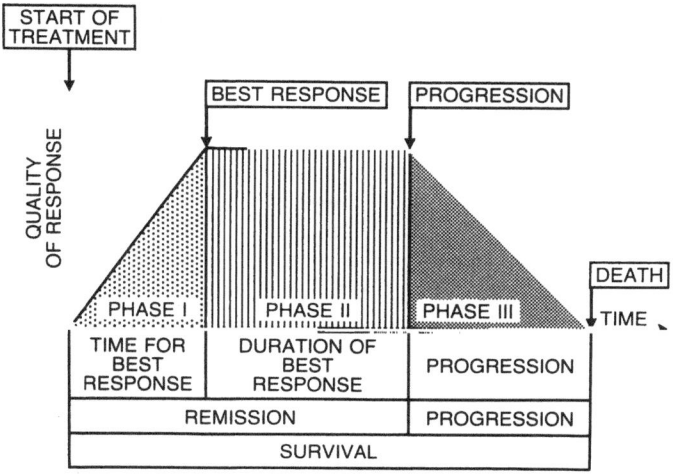

FIGURE 2 Schematic representation of the three phases of
response to treatment in advanced prostate cancer, namely
the time required to achieve the best response (phase 1),
the duration of the best response (phase 2) and the time
between progression (or relapse) and death (phase 3). The
total remission time is the sum of phases 1 and 2 while
survival includes all 3 phases between diagnosis and death.

treatment. The most striking effect is seen on complete
responses (normal bone scan and no sign or symptom of prostate
cancer) which has been observed in 49 of 186 patients (26.3%)
as compared to an average of only 4.6% in the five recent
studies limited to a blockade of testicular androgens [21, 36,
37]. The rate of complete objective response is thus increased
by 5.7-fold (p <0.01). The other striking finding is that only
6.5% of patients did not show an objective response at the
start of the combination therapy while an average of 18% of
patients failed to respond to monotherapy (orchiectomy, DES or
Leuprolide alone) in the 5 other studies, thus representing a
3-fold difference in the percentage of non-responders or
failure to treatment (p <0.01).

Figure 4 illustrates the probability of continuing
response in the total group of 186 patients who could be
evaluated. Quite remarkably, the probability is 75.4% at 1
year (117 patients), 46.2% at 2 years (61 patients) and 36.6%
at 3 years (23 patients). In contrast, the disease had
progressed before 2 years in all patients treated with
Leuprolide or DES alone [21].

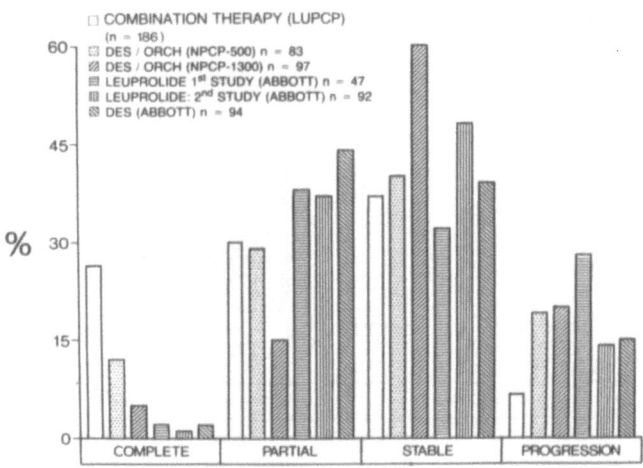

FIGURE 3 Comparison of the best objective response rates
  complete, partial, stable and progression) assessed
  according to the US NPCP cirteria following combination
  therapy with Flutamide (LUPCP) and the five comparable
  studies using orchiectomy, DES or Leuprolide alone [21,
  36, 37]. All were previously untreated patients with
  clinical stage D_2 prostate cancer.

    It is also of interest to compare the probability of
continuing response in patients who received the combination
therapy (present study) and groups of similar patients who
received DES, cyproterone acetate or medroxyprogesterone
acetate [38] (Fig. 5). Although the number of patients is
smaller while the probability after 1 year of treatment is
75.4% after combination therapy, it is reduced 60, 33 and 23%
after treatment DES, cyproterone acetate and
medroxyprogesterone acetate, respectively (Fig. 5).
    The best response achieved has an influence on the
probability of continuing response (Fig. 6). In fact, while
for complete responders, the 50% probability of continuing
response is more than 3 years, it is reduced to 630 days for
partial responders and to 517 days for stable disease. While
the difference between complete responders and any of the other
two groups is highly significant (log-rank test, p <0.0001),
there is no statistical difference between the results obtained
in patients who had a partial response and those who had stable
disease as best response.

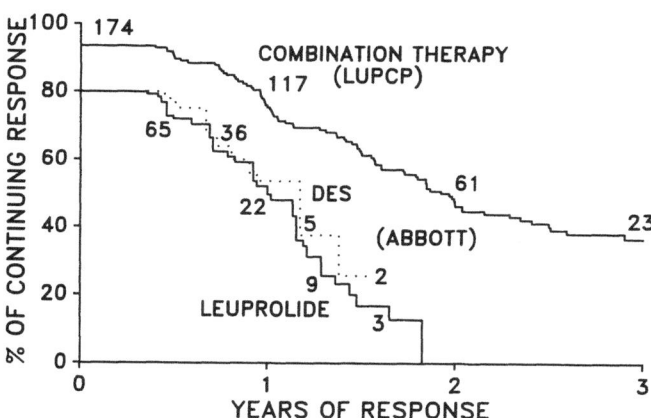

FIGURE 4 Comparison of the the probability of continuing
esponse following combination therapy (this study, (LUPCP)
and the administration of Leuprolide alone or DES [21].
The numbers on each curve correspond to the number of
patients evaluated at that time period.

While the small group of non-responders (progression) had
a median life expectancy of only 10.0 months, the best
probability of survival was obtained with the complete
responders with a 95.9% probability of survival at 3 years
(Fig. 7). Intermediate prognosis for survival was obtained for
the partial and stable categories of response. Again, while
the complete responders had a highly significant (long-rank
test, p <0.0001) better prognosis for survival than the other
groups, there was no difference between partial and stable
responders. The poor prognosis of nonresponders is highly
different (long-rank test, p <0.0001) from that of any of the
other three groups.
Following combination therapy, the probabilities of death
after 2 and 4 years are 23.8 and 51.7%, respectively, as
compared to 34 and 72%, 49 and 74% and 73 and 90% after
treatment with DES, cyproterone acetate and medroxyprogesterone
acetate, respectively [38]. The difference in death rate
following combintion therapy and the average results obtained
by monotherapy, namely DES, cyproterone acetate and
medroxyprogesterone acetate (EORTC study 30761) is better
illustrated in Fig. 9. There is an approximately
2-fold higher death rate up to 4 years of treatment in the

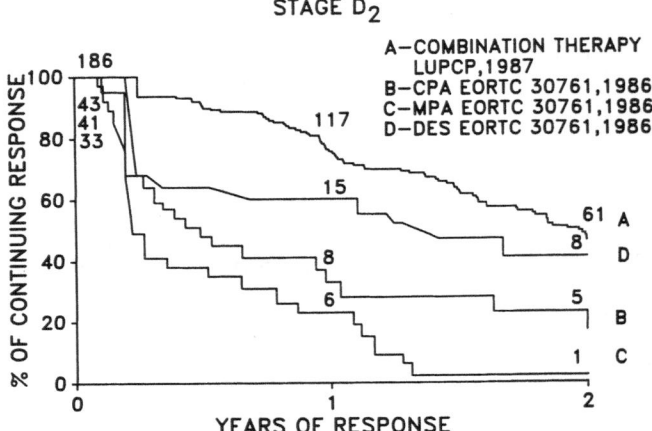

STAGE D₂

A—COMBINATION THERAPY
LUPCP,1987
B—CPA EORTC 30761,1986
C—MPA EORTC 30761,1986
D—DES EORTC 30761,1986

FIGURE 5. Comparison of the probabiliy of continuing response
following combination therapy (this study, LUPCP) and the
administration of DES, cyproterone acetate or medroxyprogesterone acetate [38]. The numbers on each curve
correspond to the number of patients evaluated at that
time period.

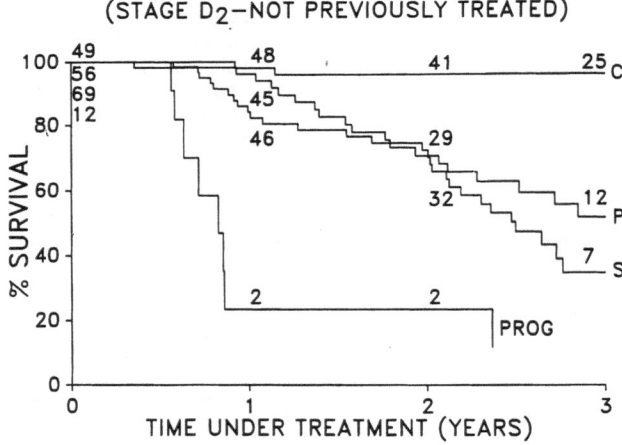

(STAGE D₂—NOT PREVIOUSLY TREATED)

FIGURE 6 Probability of continuing response according to
category of best response achieved (complete, partial or
stable) in previously untreated stage D2 patients who
received the combination therapy as first treatment.

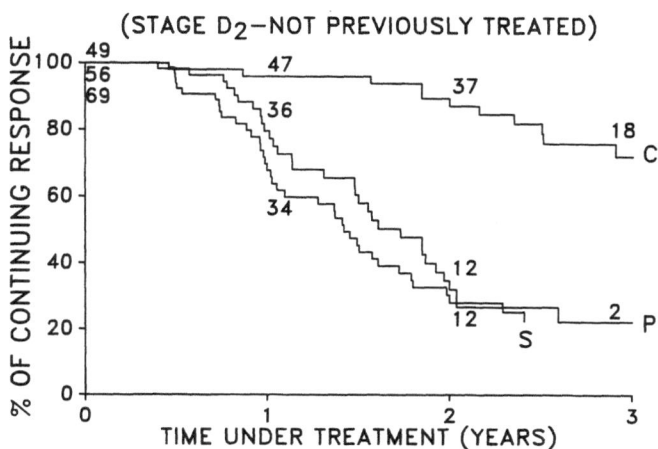

FIGURE 7 Probability of survival according to the best
objective response achieved (complete, partial, stable and
progression) in previously untreated stage D2 prostate
cancer who received the combination therapy as first
treatment.

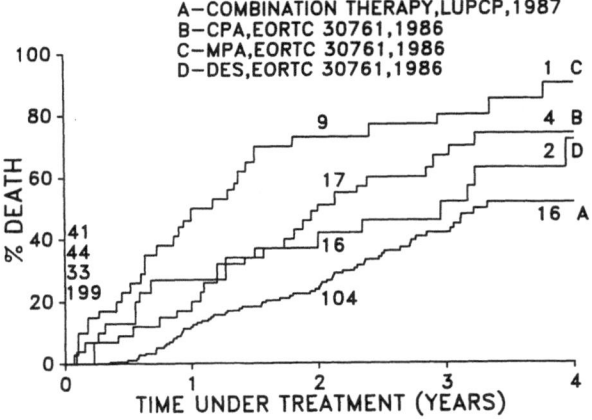

FIGURE 8 Comparison of the probability of death following
combination therapy (A) or treatment with DES (D),
cyproterone acetate (B) or medroxy progesterone acetate
(C) [38]. The numbers on each curve indicate the number
of patients alive at that time period.

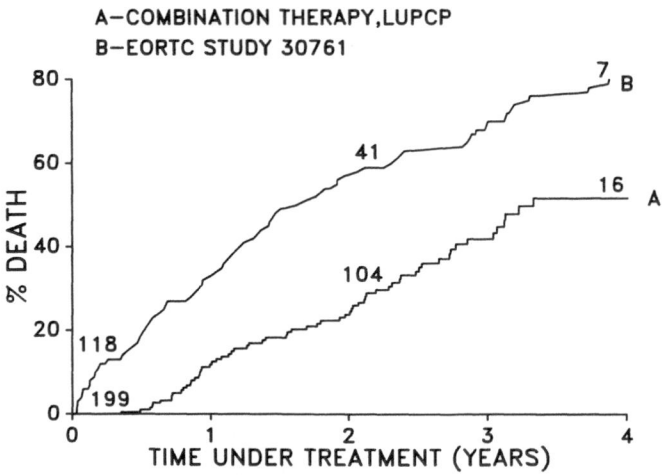

FIGURE 9   Comparison of the probability of death following
     combination therapy (A) and treatment with monotherapy
     (DES, cyproterone acetate or medroxyprogesterone acetate)
     (B).   Curve B in this figure is the sum of curves B, C and
     D in Fig. 8 [89].

EORTC study 30761 compared to our study using the combination
therapy (Fig. 9).   It should be mentioned that the death rates
presented include all causes of death, the death rate from
causes other that prostsatic cancer being approximately 5% per
year in this age group.
     Since, in most other studies, the number of patients
followed or alive after two years is usually too small, we have
used 2 years as the time for comparison of survival rates
achieved by different treatments.   23.8% of patients were dead
at 2 years of treatment with the combination therapy, an
approximately 2-fold higher death rate ranging from 40.5 to
57.4% is found in the studies where patients weere treated by
monotherapy (DES, orchiectomy or LHRH agonist alone (21, 36,
37, 40, 41, 56] (Fig. 10).
     At each visit, the patients answered a detailed question-
naire concerning any possible symtom or sign of intolerance to
the drugs.Hot flashes were described spontaneously by the
patients in approximately 50% of the cases after 1-3 months of
treatment.   Usually, the severity of the hot flashes declined
with time and disappeared within 2 years.   A loss of libido
was observed in approximately 75% of patients.   However, in 25%
of subjects, libido and potency were still present.   No
secondary effect which could not be attributed to
hypoandrogenism was observed.

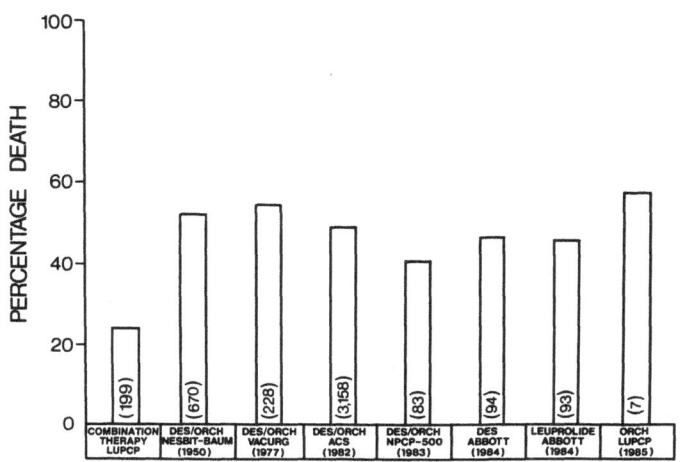

FIGURE 10 Comparison of the death rate after 2 years of
treatment with the combined androgen blockade (Laval
University Prostate Cancer Program (LUPCP) with results
obtained with standard hormonal therapies (orchiectomy
(ORCH) and/or estrogens or LHRH agonist alone) in
previously untreated stage D patients: Nesbit and Baum's
study; [39] study of the Veterans' Administration
Cooperative Urology Research Group (VACURG) [56]; survey
of the American College of Surgeons (ACS) (1982); [40] and
study 500 of the US NPCP (1983); [2] Leuprolide alone
(1984); [21, 37] and orchiectomy alone (LUPCP) (1985) (41].

COMBINATION THERAPY IN PREVIOUSLY UNTREATED STAGE C PATIENTS

Seventy men with histology-proven adenocarcinoma of the
prostate have entered into this study since September 1982,
after written informed consent. Average age at entry was 69
years (from 48 to 88 years), with a median follow-up of 666
days (62-1466). Complete clinical, urological, biochemical and
radiological evaluation of the patients was performed before
starting treatment.

All except one evaluable patients have shown a positive
response to the treatment. Moreover, only 5 patients have
shown progression or treatment failure to the combination
therapy after an average treatment period of 714 days. The
probability of survival is 98.2% and 93.7% at 1 and 2 years,

respectively. Three patients died from prostate cancer while three died from other causes (myocardial infarct, pneumonia, and suicide). All three patients had been examined at our Prostate Cancer Clinic within 6 months of death and had been found to be clinically free of disease.

Serum prostatic acid phosphatase which was elevated in forty patients before starting treatment became normal in 44, 59, 91 and 96% of them, at respectively one, two, three and six months after the beginning of combination therapy. In all except one patient, the volume of the prostate rapidly regressed and its consistency became normal during the first nine months of treatment by rectal examination. These changes were confirmed by ultrasonography of the prostate in most patients. The low urinary tract obstruction present in 3 patients was corrected by treatment. In all these patients, the transurethral catether could be removed less than 21 days after the beginning of combination therapy. Hydronephrosis originally present in eight patients disappeared in all of them before six months of therapy.

The goal of therapy in stage C prostate cancer is local control of the tumor and prolongation of the interval free of disease [42, 43]. The present data show that local control of the disease was achieved rapidly in all except one patient (98.6%).

The present data suggest that administration of the combination therapy using a pure antiandrogen (Flutamide) in association with medicasl castration ([D-Trp^6.des-Gly-NH$_2^{10}$LHRH ethylamide) at the time of diagnosis of stage C prostate cancer has advantages over standard therapies and delayed treatment [38, 44-46]. Since, in most studies, the number of patients at 3 years of treatment is too small, it seems more appropriate to use 2 years of treatment as the time of comparison.

The probability of treatment failure at 2 years of treatment with the combination therapy is only 8.2% (Fig. 11) while 24 and 32% of patients have progressed to stage D2 after radiotherapy and delayed hormonal therapy, respectively [44]. Another study [45] shows that 2 years after radiotherapy, the rate of progression to stage D2 is 18%. In a more recent study, 22% of stage C patients had progressed to stage D2 after 2 years of treatment with Estracyt or DES [46]. In another recent study, the rate of progression to stage D2 at 2 years was 40, 34 and 66% after treatment with cyproterone acetate, DES and medroxyprogesterone acetate, respectively [38]. When all the above-mentioned data of monotherapy are combined (275 patients), the rate of treatment failure is on average 28.4%, a value 3.5 higher than that observed in the present study using the well tolerated combination therapy.

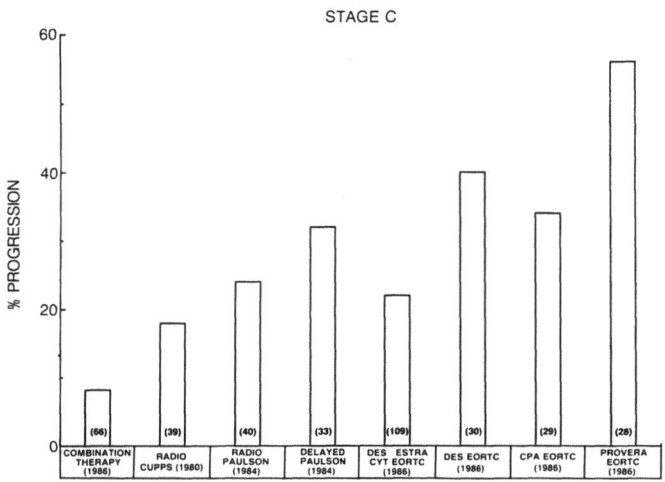

STAGE C

FIGURE 11   Comparison of the probability of treatment failure
(progression) in patients with stage C prostate cancer who
received the combination therapy (present data),
radiotherapy [44, 45], delayed treatment [44],
DES/Estracyt [46], DES [38], cyproterone acetate (CPA)
[38] or medroxyprogesterone acetate (Provera) [38].

The death rate at 2 years following the start of
combination therapy is 6.5% (Fig. 12), this value being 34% at
the same time interval following treatment with DES or estracyt
[46].   In the other EORTC study, the death rates at 2 years
after starting treatment with cyproterone acetate, DES or
medroxyprogesterone acetate were 12, 22 and 31%, respectively
[38].   When the above-mentioned data are pooled (513 patients),
the average death rate at 2 years is 22.2%.

COMBINATION THERAPY IN PATIENTS RELAPSING AFTER CASTRATION

A major problem facing the treatment of advanced prostate
cancer is the choice of therapy for patients (20 to 40% of
them) who do not respond to orchiectomy, estrogens or LHRH
agonists alone.   The same problem arises after some delay for
all the remaining 60 to 80% of patients who had an initial
response but who as a rule, show progression within 6 to 24
months.   The median life expectancy from the time of
progression is then limited to approximately 6 months [35, 47].

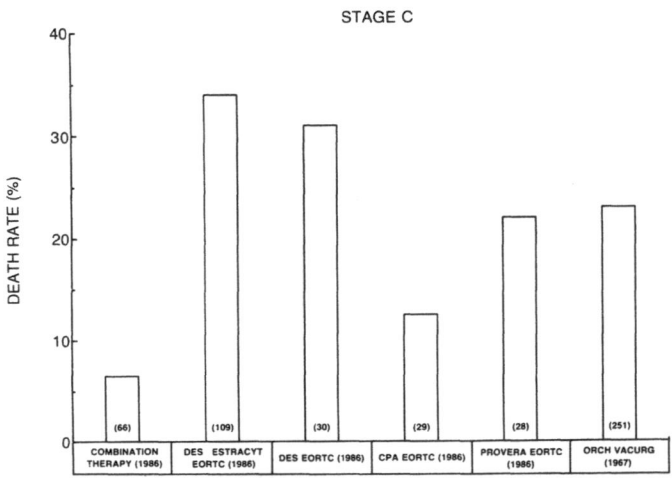

FIGURE 12   Comparison of the probability of death in patients
with clinical stage C prostate cancer who received the
combination therapy with Flutamide and the LHRH agonist
PD-Trp[6])LHRH ethylamide (present data).   DES/Estracyt
[46], DES [38], cyproterone acetate (CPA) [38], medroxyprogesterone acetate (Provera) [38] or orchiectomy [5].

Clinical evidence [48] clearly shows that
androgen-sensitive prostatic tumors remain after castration
(surgical or medical), the growth of these tumours being
stimulated by androgens of adrenal origin.   Since the aim of
all the above-mentioned therapies is to block the secretion
and/or action of adrenal androgens, a logical approach appears
to be the use of a pure antiandrogen, such as Flutamide.
The present data obtained in 209 evaluable patients show
an objective response rate (US NPCP criteria) of 35% with a
corresponding benefical effect on quality of life and survival
in the responders.   Due to its exceptionally good tolerance, it
appears that this antiandrogen should be the drug of choice to
be used in combination with castration for the treatment of
patients not responding or relapsing after castration.   The
median life expectancy is 8.1 months in the non responders,
while it is increased to more than 2.5 years in the group of
responders.
The survival rates were calculated for each group of
objective responses after combination therapy (Fig. 13).   All
the patients who have reached a complete objective response are

92

still alive. Patients who have reached partial and stable
responses show probabilities of survival at 2 years of 87 and
67%, respectively, while continuing progression of the disease
(or failure to respond objectively) leads to a 17% survival
rate at the same time interval.

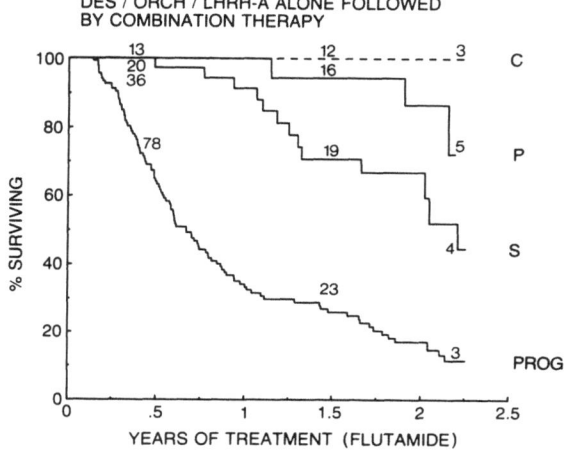

FIGURE 13 Probability of survival according to the best
objective response achieved (complete, partial, stable and
progression) following combination therapy with Flutamide
in patients who progressed after standard monotherapy.
The calculations were made starting at the time of
treatment with combination therapy. Numbers on the curve
represent the number of patients assessed or non-censored
at each period of time.

        Thus, in the largest study ever performed in a group of
patients relapsing after castration that the simple addition of
Flutamide blocks progression of the disease in as many as one
third of the patients with no or minimal side effects. The
finding of complete, partial and stable disease in respectively
6.2, 9.6 and 18.7% of the patients illustrates the important
influence of the treatment on the quality of life of these
patients. Moreover, the median life expectancy is increased.

PRETREATMENT WITH COMBINATION THERAPY BEFORE RADICAL
PROSTATECTOMY AT EARLY STAGES OF THE DISEASE

Seventeen patients (median and average age = 69 years) with
biopsy-proven prostatic carcinoma who had negative bone
scintigraphy took part in this study after written informed

consent. Bone scintigraphy was repeated twice before surgery, namely at the time of diagnosis and three months later just prior to surgery. The median follow-up of the patients after surgery is 18 months (5 to 30).

An approximately 50% atrophy of the prostatic tissues was achieved by a 3-month pretreatment of 17 patients having early stage prostatic cancer with the combination therapy. Surgical time as well as blood loss were reduced by 30 to 40%, when comparing with radical prostatectomy performed in patients not previously treated. Surgery is thus significantly facilitated, giving better chance of complete removal of cancer tissue and decreasing the occurrence of complications. The treatment was continued for a median duration of 6 months after surgery.

COMBINED ANTIANDROGEN THERAPY SHOULD NEVER BE STOPPED IN ADVANCED PROSTATE CANCER: AT THE TIME OF RELAPSE, FURTHER ANDROGEN BLOCKADE SHOULD BE ADDED

Despite the higher proportion of objective responses, the longer duration of remission, the better quality of life and the prolonged survival achieved with combination therapy [3, 10, 12, 13], delayed relapse frequently occurs and the choice of therapy becomes the main problem. Although a large series of clinical data have clearly shown that heterogeneity of androgen sensitivity is characteristic of prostate cancer [10] and fundamental observations provide an explanation for such clinical findings [49, 50], it is still common use to stop the combination therapy at the time of relapse. Such a decision is apparently based on the erroneous impression that all tumors have escaped the control of therapy and are simultaneously progressing at the time of relapse. In fact, in all cases, it is much more likely that the growth of the majority of tumors which regressed at the time of initiation of combination therapy is still blocked by the treatment and that the relapse is due to clones or tumors having androgen sensitivities different from the responding tumors.

Cessation of the combination therapy at the time of progression implies that the tumors which were kept under control by the combination therapy will start growing and add to the burden of the tumors unresponsive to combination therapy, thus leading to a more rapid progression of the disease, a poorer quality of life and earlier death. In addition to the harmful effects of the cessation of combination therapy on the evolution of prostate cancer in the individual patients, such an interruption of combination therapy at the time of relapse, invalidates the conclusions of all ongoing studies aimed at comparing the effect of combination therapy and castration alone on survival.

Since our own studies are the only ones based on the principle of optimal androgen blockade maintained at all times and where combination therapy has not been stopped at the time of relapse (aminoglutethimide + low dose hydrocortisone acetate was added), it appears useful to provide additional clinical information on this subject. A delay of 16.3 months is observed between the median time of relapse or progression of the disease under combination therapy and median survival (Fig. 14). The combination therapy was continued without interruption at the time of relapse and that further blockade

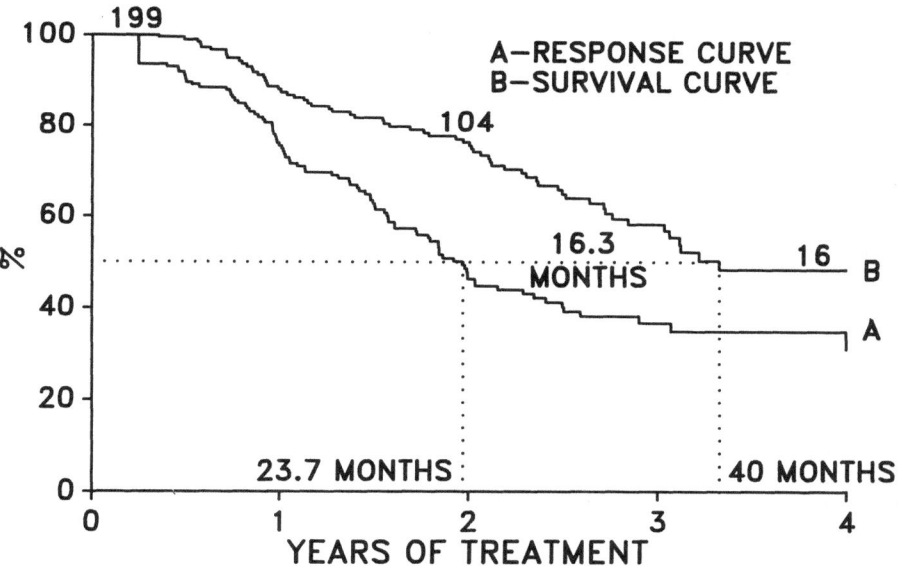

FIGURE 14 Percentage of continuing response (A) and survival (B) in 199 previously untreated stage D2 prostate cancer patients who received combination therapy as first treatment and where further blockade of adrenal androgen secretion was achieved with aminglutethimide AG, and low dose hydrocortisone acetate HC, at the time of relapse. All causes of death are included. Numbers above the lines calculated according to Kaplan-Meier [55] indicate the number of patients at that time interval.

of adrenal androgen secretion was achieved with aminoglutethimide (250mg every 8 hours) and low dose hydrocortisone acetate (10mg in the morning, 5mg in the afternoon and 5mg in the evening).

The median duration of survival observed, is longer than any other result reported so far in patients relapsing under monotherapy [6, 35, 36, 47, 51–53]. Classically, 50% of the patients (median life expectancy) are expected to die within months after first signs of relapse when first treated by castration or treatment with estrogens. In this respect, we had the opportunity to add the combination therapy to a group of 226 patients relapsing after standard monotherapy [54]. The median survival was 13.4 month (Fig. 15) or 5.3 months longer than the results obtained by the NPCP using other treatments in a similar group of patients [53]. In our study, AG+HC was added to combination therapy if no response occurred (66% of cases) or at the time of relapse to the second response (34% of patients [54]).

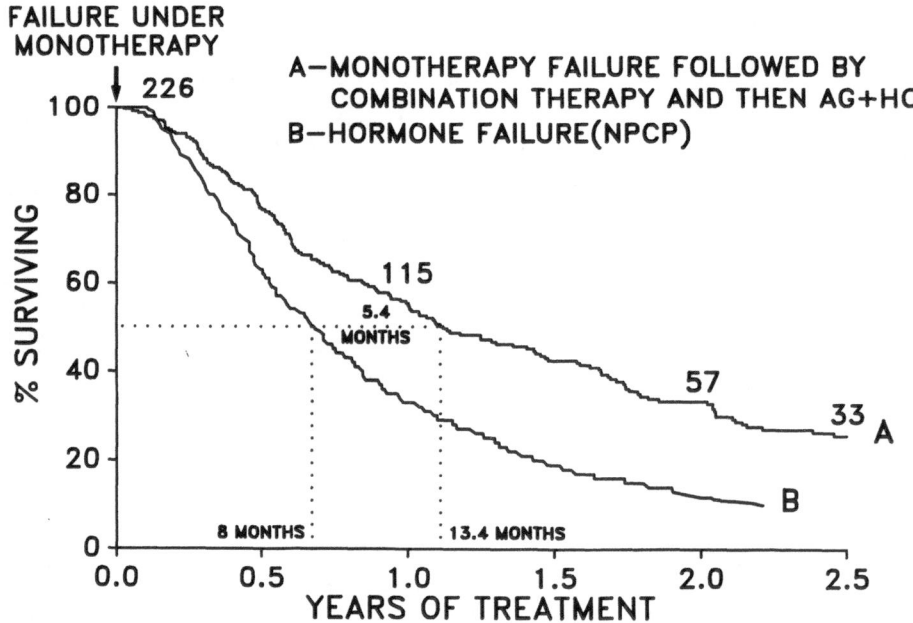

FIGURE 15 Percentage of survival in patients progressing understandard endocrine therapy (orchiectomy, estrogens or LHRH agonist alone) who received the combination therapy with Flutamide and an LHRH agonist (if not castrated) followed by AG + HC at the time of second relapse (A) compared with a study of the NPCP where a similar group of patients received various other therapies [unpublished data] (B).

When the life expectancy was calculated from time of failure under combination therapy (addition of AG+HC) in a third group of 126 patients who had previously failed to combination therapy after failure to monotherapy, the median survival was 11.0 months, a value 5.3 months shorter than that observed when the same treatment was applied in relapsing patients who received combination therapy as first treatment.

Although the present studies are not randomized, patients were assessed according to the same criteria of response [35] and minimal or no error should be expected between the groups when death is used as parameter of assessment. Since the data reported have been performed by the same group of investigators [35], the results obtained clearly indicate that starting treatment with the combination therapy does not decrease the duration of expected survival at the time of relapse. Such data strongly suggest that in addition to obtaining a longer period of remission in a larger proportion of responders, patients first treated with the combination therapy live longer after progression of the disease than patients who progress after monotherapy received as initial treatment. Maximal survival, however, requires continuation of optimal androgen blockade until the last day of life. The drugs presently available to achieve the proposed androgen blockade are well or extremely well tolerated, thus permitting the maximal benefits described above without affecting the quality of life.

REFERENCES

1.   CA-A Cancer Journal for Clinicians (1987). Amer Cancer Soc, p.37
2.   Huggins, C and Hodges, CV (1941). Studies on prostatic cancer. I. Effect of castration, of estrogen and of androgen injection on serum phosphatases in metastatic carcinoma of the prostate. Cancer Res, 1, 293
3.   Labrie, F, Dupont, A and Belanger, A (1985). A complete blockade for the treatment of prostate cancer. In: De Vita, VT, Hellman, S and Rosenberg, SA (eds.) "Important Advances in Oncology". p.193. (Philadelphia: J.B. Lippincott)
4.   Glashan, RW and Robinson, MRG (1981). Cardiovascular complications in the treatment of prostatic carcinoma. Brit J Urol, 53, 624
5.   Veterans Administration Cooperative Urological Research Group (1967). Carcinoma of the prostate. Treatment comparisons. J Urol, 98, 516
6.   Johansson, JE, Andersson, SO, Beckman, KW, Lingardh, G and Zador, G (1987). Clincal evaluation of Flutamide and estramustine as initial treatment of metastatic carcinoma of the prostate. Urology, 29, 55

7.   Labrie, F, Belanger, A, Cusan, L, Seguin, C, Pelletier, G, Kelly, PA, Lefebvre, FA, Lemay, A and Raynaud, JP (1980). Antifertility effects of LHRH agonists in the male. J Androl, 1, 209

8.   Labrie, F, Dupont, A, Belanger, A, Lachance, R and Giguere, M (1985). Long-term treatment with luteinizing hormone-releasing hormone agonists and maintenance of serum testosterone to castration concentrations. Brit Med J, 291, 369

9.   Pike, A, Peeling, WB, Harper, ME, Pierrepoint, CG and Griffiths, K (1970). Testosterone metabolism in vivo by human prostatic tissue. Biochem J, 120, 443

10.   Labrie, F, Dupont, A and Belanger, A (1987). LHRH agonists and antiandrogens in prostate cancer. In: Ratliff, TL and Catalona, WJ (eds.) "Genitourinary Cancer". p.157. (Boston: Martinus Nijhoff)

11.   Labrie, F, Dupont, A, Belanger, A, Cusan, L, Lacourciere, Y, Monfette, G, Laberge, JG, Emond, JP, Fazekas, ATA, Raynaud, JP and Husson, JM (1982). New hormonal therapy in prostatic carcinoma: combined treatment with an LHRH agonist and an antiandrogen. Clin Invest Med, 5, 267

12.   Ojasso, T (1987). Nilutamide. Drugs of the Future, 12, 763

13.   Moguilewsky, M, Fiet, J, Tournemine, C and Raynaud, JP (1986). Pharmacology of an antiandrogen, Anandron, used as an adjuvant therapy in the treatment of prostate cancer. J Steroid Biochem, 24, 139

14.   Labrie, F, Dupont, A, Belanger, A and Lachance, R (1987). Flutamide eliminates the risk of disease flare in prostatic cancer patients treated with a luteinizing hormone-releasing hormone agonist. J Urol, 138, 804

15.   Faure, N, Labrie, F, Lemay, A, Belanger, A, Gourdeau, Y, Laroche, B and Robert, G (1982). Inhibition of serum androgen levels by chronic intranasal and subcutaneous administration of a potent luteinizing hormone-releasing hormone (LH-RH) agonist in adult men. Fertil Steril, 37, 416

16.   Allen, JM, O'Shea, JM, Mashiter, K, Williams, G and Bloom, SR (1983). Advanced carcinoma of the prostate: treatment with a gonadotrophin releasing hormone agonist. Brit Med J, 286, 1607

17.   Walker, KJ, Nicholson, RI, Turkes, AO, Turkes, A, Griffiths, K, Robinson, M, Crispen, Z and Dris, S (1983). Therapeutic potential of the LHRH agonist, ICI 118630, in the treatment of advanced prostatic carcinoma. Lancet, 2, 413

18.   Waxman, JH, Wass, JAH, Hendry, WF, Whitfield, HN, Besser, GM, Malpas, JS and Oliver, RTD (1983). Treatment with gonadotrophin releasing hormone analogue in advanced prostatic cancer. Brit Med J, 286, 1309

19.   Wenderoth, UK and Jacobi, GH (1984). Three years of experience with the GnRH-analogue buserelin in 100 patients with advanced prostatic cancer. In: Labrie, R, Belanger, A and Dupont, A (eds.) "LHRH and its analogues: Basic and Clinical Aspects". p.349. (New York: Excerpta Medica)

20.   Kahan, A, Delrieu, F, Amor, B, Chiche, R and Steg, A
(1984). Disease flare induced by D-Trp[6]-LHRH analogue in
patients with metastatic prostatic cancer. Lancet, 1, 971
21.   The Leuprolide Study Group (1984). Leuprolide versus
diethylstilbestrol for metastatic prostate cancer. New Engl J
Med, 311, 1281
22.   Waxman, JH, Man, A, Hendry, WF, Whitfield, HN, Besser,
GM, Tiptaff, RC, Paris, AMI and Oliver, RTD (1985). Importance
of early tumour exacerbation in patients treated with
long-acting analogues of gonadotrophin releasing hormone for
advanced prostatic cancer. Brit Med J. 291, 1387
23.   St-Arnaud, R, Lachance, R, Dupont, A and Labrie, F
(1986). Serum luteinizing hormone (LH) biological activity in
castrated patients with cancer of the prostate receiving a pure
antiandrogen and in estrogen-pretreated patients treated with
an LH-releasing hormone agonist and antiandrogen. J Clin Endocr
Metab, 63, 297
24.   Labrie, F, Dupont, A, Belanger, A, St-Arnaud, R, Giguere,
M, Lacourciere, Y, Emond, J and Monfette, G (1986). Treatment
of prostate cancer with gonadotropin-releasing hormone
agonists. Endocr Rev, 7, 67
25.   Neri, R, Florance, K, Koziol, P and Van Cleave, S
(1972). A biological profile of a nonsteroidal antiandrogen,
SCH13521 (4'-nitro-3'trifluoromethylisobutyranilide).
Endocrinology, 91, 427
26.   Simard, J, Luthy, I, Guay, J, Belanger, A and Labrie, F
(1986). Characteristics and interaction of the antiandrogen
flutamide with the androgen receptor in various target
tissues. Mol Cell Endocrinol, 44, 261
27.   Belanger, A, Brochu, M and Cliche, J (1986). Levels of
plasma steroid glucuronides in intact and castrated men with
prostate cancer. J Clin Endocrinol Metab, 62, 812
28.   Labrie, F, Luthy, I, Veilleux, R, Simard, J, Belanger, A
and Dupont, A (1987). New concepts on the androgen sensitivity
of prostate cancer. In: Murphy, G (ed.) "Second Int Symp on
Prostate Cancer". p.145. (New York: Alan R. Liss)
29.   Murray, R and Pitt, P (1985). Treatment of advanced
prostatic cancer resistant to conventional therapy with
aminoglutethimide. Eur J Cancer Clin Oncol, 21, 453
30. Maddy, JA, Winternitz, WW and Norrell, H (1971).
Cryohypophysectomy in the management of advanced prostatic
cancer. Cancer, 28, 322
31.   Becker, H (1986). Endocrine treatment of advanced
prostate cancer. 14th Int Cancer Cong, Budapest, abstract #3291
32.   Drago, JR, Santen, RJ, Lipton, A, Worgul, TJ, Harvey, HA,
Boucher, A, Manni, A and Rohner, TJ (1984). Clinical effect of
aminoglutethimide, medical adrenalectomy, in treatment of 43
patients with advanced prostatic carcinoma. Cancer, 953, 1447
33.   Kreis, W, Ahmann, FR and Crawford, ED (1986). Clinical
effects and hormone profiles in men with advanced prostate
cancer under treatment with aminoglutethimide. 14th Int Cancer
Congr, Budapest, abstract #4619

34.   Stoliar, B and Albert, PJ (1974). SCH13521 in the
treatment of advanced carcinoma of the prostate. J Urol, 111,
803
35.   Slack, NH, Brady, MF, Murphy, GP and Investigators in the
National Prostatic Cancer Project (1984). Stable versus
partial response in advanced prostate cancer. The Prostate, 4,
401
36.   Murphy, GP, Beckley, S, Brady, MF, Chu, M, Dekernion, JB,
Dhabuwala, C, Gaeta, JF, Gibbons, RP, Loening, SA, McKiel, CF,
McLeod, DG, Pontes, JE, Prout, GR, Scardino, PT, Schlegel, JU,
Schmidt, JD, Scott, WW, Slack, NH and Soloway, M (1983).
Treatment of newly diagnosed metastatic prostate cancer
patients with chemotherapy agents in combination with hormones
versus hormones alone. Cancer, 51, 1264
37.   Smith, JA, Glode, LM, Wettlaufer, JN, Stein, BS, Glass,
AG, max, TD, Anbar, D, Jagst, CL and Murphy, GP (1985).
Clinical effects of gonadotropin-releasing hormone analogue in
metastatic carcinoma of the prostate. Urology, 20, 106
38.   Pavone-Macaluso, M, De Voogt, HJ, Viggiano, G, Baqrasolo,
E, Lardennois, B, De Pauw, M and Sylvester, R (1986).
Comparison of diethylstilbestrol, cyproterone acetate and
medroxyprogesterone acetate in the treatment of advanced
prostatic cancer: final analysis of a randomized phase III
trial of the European Organization for Research on Treatment of
Cancer Urological Group. J Urol, 136, 624
39.   Mesbit, RM and Baum, WC (1950). Endocrine control of
prostatic carcinoma: clinical and statistical survey of 1,818
cases. JAMA, 143, 1317
40.   Mettlin, C, Natarajan, N and Murphy, GP (1982). Recent
paOterns of care of prostatic cancer patients in the United
States: results from the surveys of the American College of
Surgeons Commission on Cancer. Int Adv Sur Oncol, 5, 277
41.   Labrie, F, Dupont, A, Belanger, A, Lachance, R and
Giguere, M\(1985). Long-term treatment with luteinzing
hormone-releasing hormone agonists and maintenance of serum
testosterone to castration concentrations. Brit Med J, 291, 369
42.   Gibbons, RP, Mason, JT, Correa, RA Jr, Cummings, KB,
Taylor, WJ, Hafermann, MD and Richardson, RD (1979). Carcinoma
of the prostate: local control with external beam radiation
therapy. J. Urol, 121, 310
43.   Tomlinson, RL, Currie, DP and Boyce, WH (1977). Radical
prostatectomy: palliation for stage C carcinoma of the
prostate. J Urol, 117, 85
44.   Paulson, DF (1984). Treatment of locally confined
prostatic cancer: radiotherapy versus surgery-limits of
curability. In: Kurth, KIH, Debryene, FMJ, Schraeder, FH,
Splinter, TAW, Wagener, TDJ (eds.) "Progress and Controversies
in Oncological Urology" p.482. (New York: Alan R. Liss)
45.   Cupps, RE, Utz, DC, Fleming, TR, Carson, CC, Bastable,
JRG, Glashan, RW, Bouffioux, C, Lardennois, B, Williams, RE, De
Pauw, M and Sylvester, R (1980). Definitive ratiation therapy
for prostatic carcinoma: Mayo Clinic Experience. J Uro, 124,
855

46.   Smith, PD., Suciu, S, Robinson, MRG, Richards, B,
Bastable, JRG, Glashan, RW, Bouffioux, C, Lardennois, B,
Williams, RE, De Pauw, M and Sylvester, R (1986). A comparison
of the effectiveness of diethylstilbestrol with low dose
estramustine phosphate in the treatment of advanced prostatic
cancer: final analysis of a phase III trial of the European
Organization for Research on Treatment of Cancer. J Urol, 136,
619
47.   Johnson, DE, Scott, WW, Gibbsons, RP, Prout, GR, Schmidt,
JD, Chu, TM, Gaeta, J, Sarott, J and Murphy, GP (1977).
National randomized study of chemotherapeutic agents in
advanced prostatic carcinoma: progress report. Cancer Treat
Rep, 61, 317
48.   Higgins, C and Scott, WW (1945). Bilateral adrenalectomy
in prostatic cancer. Ann Sur, 122, 1031
49.   Labrie, F and Veilleux, R (1986). A wide range of
sensitivities to androgens develops in cloned Shionogi mouse
mammary tumor cells. The Prostate, 8, 293
50.   Luthy, I and Labrie, F (1987). Development of androgen
resistance in mouse mammary tumor cells can be prevented by the
antiandrogen flutamide. The Prostate, 10, 89
51.   Sogani, PC, Ray, B and Whitmore, WF Jr (1975). Advanced
prostatic carcinoma: flutamide therapy after conventional
endocrine treatment. Urology, 6, 164
52.   Whitmore, WF Jr (1973). The natural history of prostatic
cancer. Cancer, 32, 1104
53.   Brendler, H (1959). Current cancer concepts: therapy
with orchiectomy or estrogens or both. JAMA, 210, 1074
54.   Labrie, F, Dupont, A, Giguere, M, Borsanyi, JP,
Lacourciere, Y, Monfette, G, Edmond, J and Bergeron, N (1988).
Benefits of combination therapy with Flutamide in patients
relapsing after castration. Brit J Urol, 61, (in press)
55.   Kaplan, EL and Meier, P (1958). Non parametric
estimation from incomplete observation. Amer Statist Assoc J,
457
56.   Jordan, WP Jr, Blackard, CE and Byar, DP (1977).
Reconsideration of orchiectomy in the treatment of advanced
prostatic carcinoma. South Med J, 70, 1411

10

MEDICAL VERSUS SURGICAL ORCHIECTOMY IN ADVANCED PROSTATIC CANCER

H. PARMAR, R.H. PHILLIPS, L. EDWARDS and **S.L. LIGHTMAN**
Charing Cross and Westminster Medical School,
and Westminster Hospital, London

INTRODUCTION

There are now several potent agonist analogues of GnRH which exert inhibitory effects on the pituitary gonadal axis [1-5]. [D-Trp^6]LHRH and other GnRH agonists have an excellent safety profile and are proving to be useful in both benign and malignant disease [6-8]. Long-term administration of these analogues results in down-regulation of GnRH receptors and subsequent decrease in gonadotrophin secretion. This fall in gonadotrophins is accompanied by a reduction in gonadal steroidogenesis (medical orchiectomy). This is the predominant mechanism by which [D-Trp^6]LHRH has a beneficial effect in prostatic cancer, although additional mechanisms may also be of importance.

Most of the analogues require daily administration either subcutaneously or intra-nasally. We here report results of a prospective randomised trial comparing the efficacy and safety of a slow-release preparation of [D-Trp^6]LHRH microcapsules, given monthly, compared with orchiectomy as first line treatment of advanced prostatic cancer.

METHODS

Study design

The study was conducted in six centres in South-East England. Entry and exclusion criteria are given in Table 1. All centres had ethical committee approval and the patients were selected by a balanced randomisation schedule stratified for centre and clinical investigator. Informed consent was obtained in all patients. Withdrawal from the assigned group or treatment was only effected after tumour progression. Criteria for tumour response are given in Table 2. No complete response category has been included in our study since hormonal treatments are not associated with clinical cure and since this category is generally considered misleading in cancer treatment using hormones.

Table 1. Criteria for patient selection

Entry Criteria
   a) Histologically proven prostatic cancer
   b) Expected survival >3 months
   c) Bone metastases
   d) Lymph node metastases outside the pelvis
   e) Metastases to other soft tissues except the
      brain
   f) No previous chemotherapy, hormone therapy or
      radiotherapy

Exclusion Criteria
   a) Life threatening renal, liver, cardiac or
      malignant disease

Investigations and follow-up

Patients were assessed by clinical examination at monthly
intervals for 3 months and thereafter at 3-monthly intervals for 2
years. At each follow-up blood samples were taken for full blood
count, urea and electrolytes, liver function tests, calcium,
phosphate, proteins, LH, FSH, prolactin, testosterone and
prostatic acid phosphatase (PAP). LH, FSH, prolactin,
testosterone and PAP were measured by radioimmunoassay at
Westminster Hospital. Regular isotope bone scans, radiographs of
chest and pelvis, serial radiographs of sites of metastases,
transabdominal ultrasound scan of prostate and, if indicated and
available, lymphangiography and computed tomographic (CT) scans of
the abdomen and pelvis were carried out. Pain and cross-validated
psychological questionnaires [9-11] were administered before and
after treatment. Patients on [D-Trp6]LHRH were assessed on
day 8, to evaluate the possibility of tumour flare, and monthly
thereafter. Karnofsky performance status was assessed before and
after starting treatment at 3 monthly intervals. Patients on
[D-Trp6]LHRH at Westminster hospital had GnRH tests at 6-monthly
intervals, just prior to the monthly injection, to evaluate
hormonal escape.

Treatment protocol

The [D-Trp6]LHRH injections were given on day 1, day 8, day 28
and thereafter once a month. Paients randomised for surgery had
bilateral orchiectomy and synthetic implants were inserted in some
patients at the time of operation. Patients remained in the
assigned group until tumour progression. After progression some
patients in the surgical orchiectomy group were given monthly
[D-Trp6]LHRH to assess whether or not gonadotrophins were
trophic for prostatic cancer growth.

Table 2. Criteria of objective clinical responses

Response	Tumour Masses	Prostatic Acid Phosphatase	Osteoblastic Lesions	Osteolytic Lesions	Weight, Symptoms Performance Status
Partial (all, if present)	>50% reduction of at least one mass	Normalised	No progression	Recalcification of some	No deterioration
Objective stable (all, if present)	No increase in size >25% no new lesions	Decrease but not to normal	Stable	Not worse	No deterioration
Progressive (any of following)	Increase in size >25%; new lesion	Increase by 50% over previous level	Increase in size and/or no. of metastases	Increase in size and/or no. of metastases	Deterioration

Statistical methods

All the biochemical, hormonal, PAP and psychological data were
analysed using the Mann-Whitney U test. The Friedman analysis of
variance was used to assess the hormonal and PAP data within each
group. The chi-squared test was used to assess clinical objective
response and the logrank test to assess the survival data. All
the p values quoted are two-tailed.

RESULTS

All pre-treatment patient characteristics examined for both groups
were similar and there was no statistical difference between the
groups. Fifty-eight patients were randomised to medical
orchiectomy and 55 to surgical orchiectomy. Three patients were
excluded from analysis from the [D-Trp[6]]LHRH group and 6 from
the orchiectomy group. Two patients in the [D-Trp[6]]LHRH only
received the drug at 3 monthly intervals and one died from a road

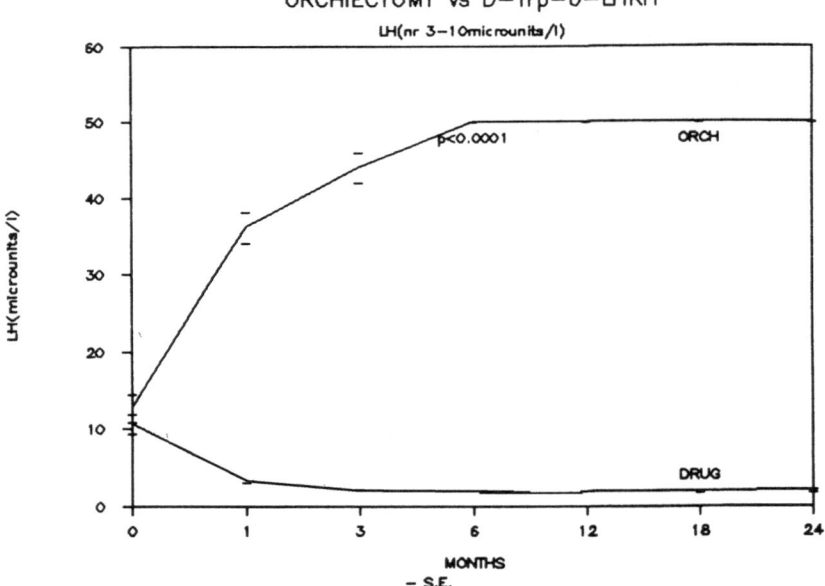

FIGURE 1 LH response for orchiectomy and [D-Trp[6]]LHRH

traffic accident at 3 months. Of the six patients excluded from
the orchiectomy group, two refused orchiectomy, 2 had treatment
prior to orchiectomy, 1 died at three weeks from a myocardial
infarction and 1 failed to attend for follow-up. Hormonal and PAP
responses in all evaluable patients to orchiectomy and
[D-Trp[6]]LHRH are shown in Figs. 1-5. In the [D-Trp[6]]LHRH

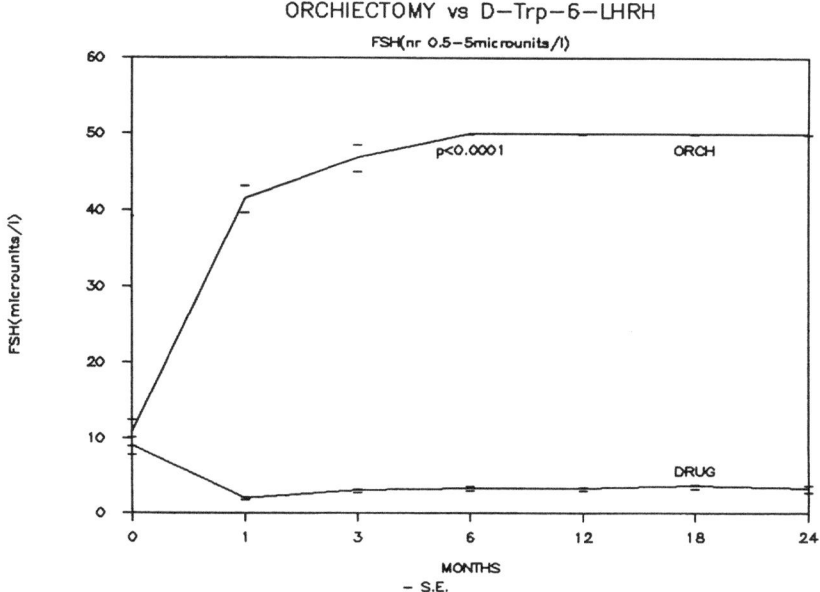

FIGURE 2 FSH response for orchiectomy and [D-Trp⁶]LHRH

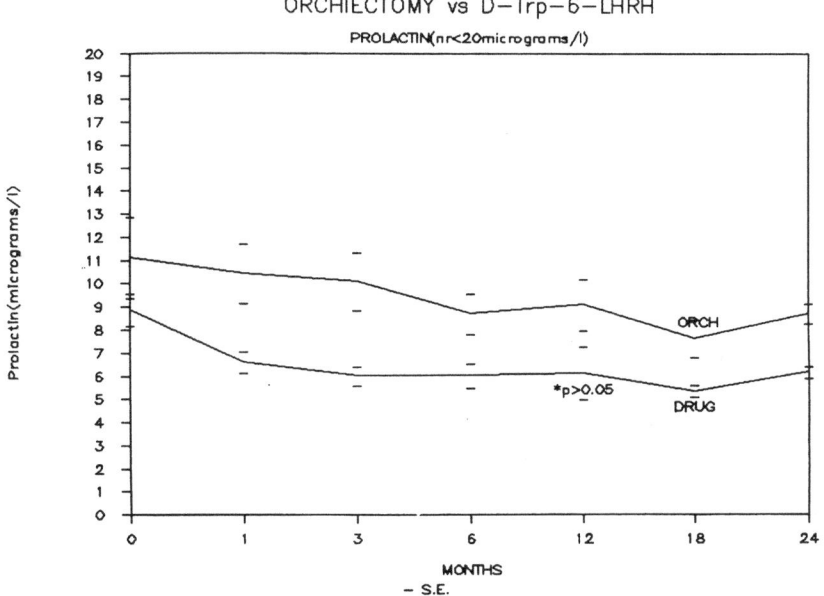

FIGURE 3 Prolactin response for orchiectomy and [D-Trp⁶]LHRH

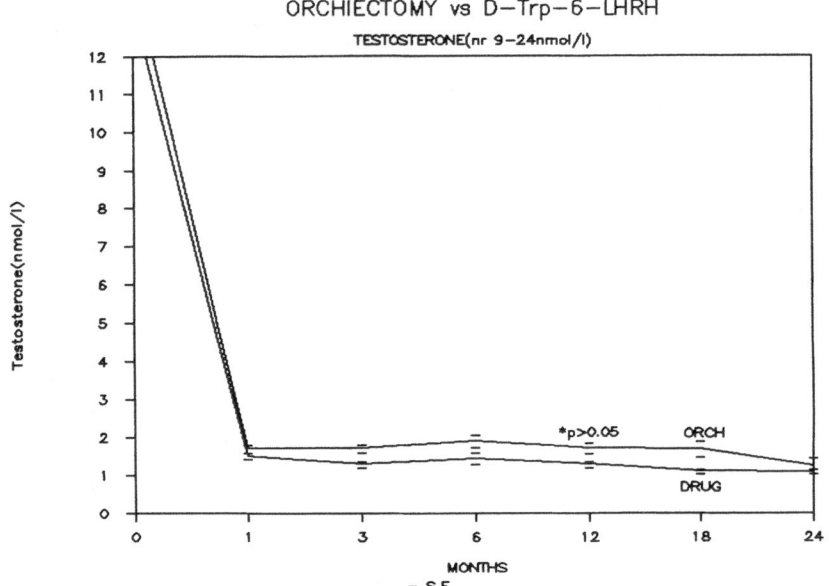

FIGURE 4 Testosterone response for orchiectomy and [D-Trp[6]]LHRH

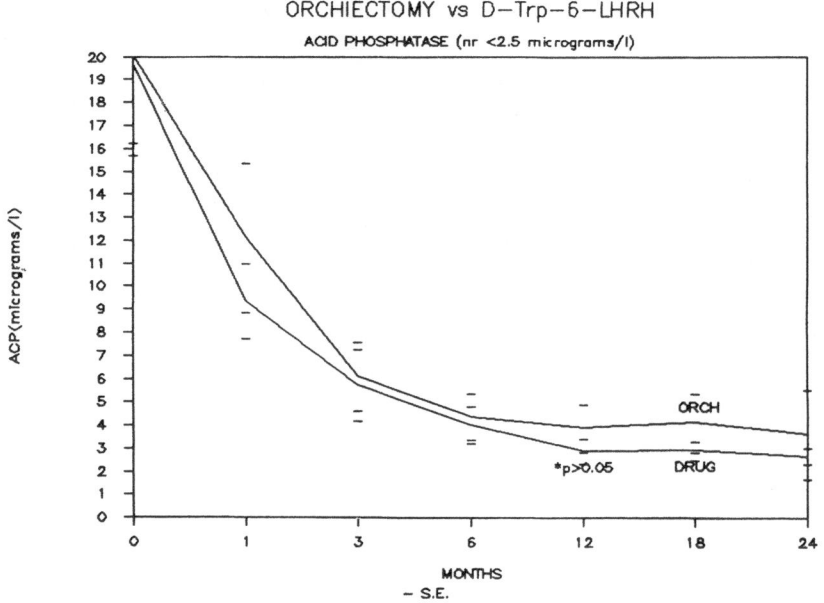

FIGURE 5 Acid phosphatase response for orchiectomy and
           [D-Trp[6]]LHRH

group at one month or later gonadotrophins were significantly
suppressed while in the surgical orchiectomy group LH and FSH were
grossly elevated. This difference was highly significant
(p<0.0001) and was maintained for the entire duration of the
study. Plasma testosterone levels decreased significantly in both
groups but there was no statistical difference between the groups
at one month or later. Castrate levels of testosterone were
maintained in both groups for the entire duration of the study.
There was no difference between the groups in the levels of PAP
before or after treatment although there was a significant drop
within each group (p<0.05). Results of the GnRH tests carried out
at six monthly intervals just prior to the monthly injection are
shown in Tables 3 and 4; gonadotrophin response was normal before
starting treatment and was significantly suppressed at 6, 12, 18
and 24 mths (p=0.002).

Table 3. LH response to GnRH tests

| Time | LH | | |
(months)	0 mins	20 mins	60 mins
0	8.0±0.68	20.70±3.50	22.80±3.50
6	2.5±0.21	2.60±0.23	2.50±0.24
12	2.7±0.12	2.83±0.16	2.68±0.17
18	2.7±0.14	2.90±0.17	2.73±0.16
24	2.6±0.15	2.70±0.16	2.71±0.16

Table 4. FSH response to GnRH tests

| Time | FSH | | |
(months)	0 mins	20 mins	60 mins
0	8.83±1.71	12.10±2.04	14.80±2.60
6	2.54±0.49	2.65±0.46	2.65±0.43
12	3.03±0.32	3.26±0.33	3.19±0.34
18	3.20±0.33	3.04±0.33	3.20±0.33
22	3.30±0.32	3.40±0.33	3.40±0.34

Twenty-six patients out of 34 in the [D-Trp[6]]LHRH group
and 24 out of 31 in the orchiectomy group had improvement in
urinary symptoms at 3 months (Table 5). Two patients from both
groups required transurethral resection of prostate (T.U.R.P.).
Five patients with urinary retention improved after treatment with
[D-Trp[6]]LHRH and 2 improved after orchiectomy. Three patients

109

Table 5. Symptoms, performance and metastatic results of the trial

Criterion	[D-Trp^6]LHRH	Orchiectomy
Urinary symptoms		
On entry	34	31
Improved	26(76%)	24(77%)
Stable	6(18%)	5(16%)
T.U.R.P.	2(6%)	2(7%)
Urinary retention		
On entry	8	6
Improved	5(63%)	2(33%)
T.U.R.P.	3(37%)	4(66%)
Pain		
On entry	40	36
Improved	34(85%)	30(83%)
Worse	6(15%)	6(17%)
Performance status		
On entry	55	49
Improved Karnofsky	34(62%)	28(57%)
Metastases		
On entry	51	44
Improved	18(35%)	14(32%)
Stable	25(49%)	21(48%)
Worse	8(16%)	9(20%)

with urinary retention in the [D-Trp^6]LHRH group and 4 in the orchiectomy group required T.U.R.P. Pain score improved in 85% of patients in the [D-Trp^6]LHRH group and 83% of patients in the orchiectomy group. Six patients in both groups had deterioration in pain symptoms. Thirtyfive percent of patients in the [D-Trp^6]LHRH group and 32% in the orhiectomy group had disappearance or improvement in one or more metastases at 3 months. Sixteen percent of [D-Trp^6]LHRH patients and 20% of orchiectomy patients had evidence of new metastases at 3 months. Those patients that failed to respond to treatment with surgical orchiectomy and those that progressed after initial response were subsequently treated with [D-Trp^6]LHRH. Twenty four patients were treated in this way. Only 1 patient achieved partial remission and 4 were assessed to have stable disease; significant gonadotrophin suppression (p<0.0001) was achieved in all patients treated as a second line with [D-Trp^6]LHRH. There was no significant change in plasma testosterone and no correlation of response with changes in hormonal status in these patients.

Side effects

There were no reports of any local reaction around the injection site and the patients experienced only mild discomfort on administration, which subsided within a few minutes to a few hours. Seventysix percent of patients on [D-Trp^6]LHRH and 73% of patients in the orchiectomy group experienced vasomotor flushing. There was no statistical difference between the groups for the average number of attacks of flushing and the subjective severity. Forty-two patients in the [D-Trp^6]LHRH group and 44 patients in the orchiectomy group had decreased libido or impotence. However most of the patients were not sexually active either prior to or after starting treatment. There was no incidence of gynaecomastia noted in either group and no patient had any cardiovascular symptoms attributable to either treatment. There was a subjective decrease in size of the testes noted in most of the patients started on [D-Trp^6]LHRH, but only a few patients mentioned it and no actual measurements were taken.

Three patients in the [D-Trp^6]LHRH group experienced a disease flare between day 1 and day 10. This was manifested by gross lymphoedema of the legs in one patient and increased pain in the others. The flare symptoms completely subsided in all patients by 8 weeks of treatment. No patients experienced any further flares on any subsequent injection once down regulation of the pituitary gonadal axis was established.

Psychological effects

The psychological questionaire was analysed and broken down into its various parameters. There was no difference noted pre-treatment between the groups for anxiety, depression, cheerfulness, fatigue, energy, anger, composure or thoughtfulness. At 6 months in the [D-Trp^6]LHRH group there was a trend to less fatigue, anger, composure, depression and anxiety. This was also associated with increased cheerfulness and energy when comparing the medical versus surgical orchiectomy group. However these results are not statistically significant by the Mann-Whitney U test.

OVERALL RESPONSE

The responses of all evaluable patients at 12 weeks or later are shown in Table 3. There was no statistically significant difference between the 2 groups in clinical objective response, tumour progression or survival. Twenty-eight patients died in the [D-Trp^6]LHRH group (mean survival 16 months) and 25 patients died in the orchiectomy group (mean survival 18 months). A survival graph of all evaluable patients up to 45 months is shown in Fig. 6.

Table 6. Overall response of evaluable patients

Response	[D-Trp⁶]LHRH	Orchiectomy
Partial	20(36%)	16(33%0
Stable	26(47%)	24(49%)
Progressive	9(16%)	9(18%)
Mean survival	16 months	18 months

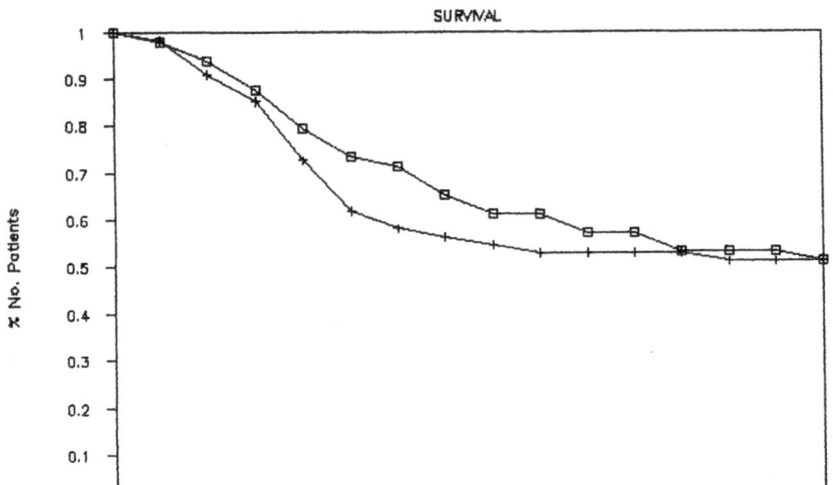

FIGURE 6 Survival data for orchiectomy and [D-Trp⁶]LHRH patients.

DISCUSSION

Ever since 1941 following the famous studies of Huggins and
Hodges, orchiectomy and/or oestrogens have been the major
therapies available for advanced prostatic cancer [12-13].
Ostrogens are associated with cardio-vascular toxicity while
orchiectomy has an adverse psychological impact on patients [14].
Many clinicians regard orchiectomy as the initial treatment of
choice in the management of advanced prostatic cancer [15-16].
Therefore we felt it prudent to test medical orchiectomy using
[D-Trp⁶]LHRH against surgical orchiectomy.

Our data show continued long term suppression of serum gonadotrophin levels in patients treated with [D-Trp[6]]LHRH. Following surgical orchiectomy the FSH and LH levels were >40 units per litre and remained at this level for the entire duration of the study. Whether this difference in gonadotrophin secretion is of any importance is not known but gonadotrophins have been implicated as trophic factors for prostatic cancer growth [17]. Indeed hypophysectomy has been shown to produce subjective and objective remissions in relapsed advanced prostatic cancer [18]. Clearly this study demonstrates that the difference in secretion of gonadotrophins between the groups is not clinically significant as far as response and suvival are concerned. Indeed most patients in the relasped surgical orchiectomy group with high gonadotrophin levels failed to respond to subsequent treatment with [D-Trp[6]]LHRH. Therefore we do not feel that gonadotrophins can be regarded as trophic factors for prostatic cancer growth, although it is possible these patients had developed hormone resistant tumours at this stage as a direct result of selecting out hormone resistant clones following orchiectomy. However this argument mainly applies to testosterone since these patients were only deprived of this hormone at the start of treatment.

We achieved a minor reduction of prolactin in both groups. Prolactin potentiates androgen activity in the prostate [19] and its reduction may be beneficial in some patients [20]. It seems unlikely that this small reduction in prolactin is contributing directly to the tumour response. It is interesting to note, however, that elevated levels of prolactin may be associated with a poor prognosis [21]. It this is the case then any treatment that could increase the levels of prolactin should be avoided. Oestrogens, apart from causing increased cardiovascular toxicity, gynaecomastia, depression and fluid retention, also elevate levels of prolactin. This is a further reason for avoiding oestrogens as a primary treatment of prostatic cancer when other equally effective treatments are available [22].

Although sexual function declines with age, approximately 50% of males aged 70-89 yrs are sexually active [23]. All forms of treatment of prostatic cancer have been reported to cause sexual dysfunction. Erectile dysfunction has been reported in 6 to 90% of patients treated with radiotherapy, oestrogens, orchiectomy, antiandrogens and gonadotrophin releasing hormone agonists [23-25]. Sexual dysfunction figures as high as 84% have been reported even for external beam radiation [26]. It is clear that any treatment that reduces the level of testosterone is likely to cause diminished libido and impotence.

The psychological effects of treatment for cancer tend to be ignored or underemphasised in most studies but are undoubtedly of great importance to the patient in his struggle against the disease. This study shows a slightly decreased but statistically non-significant psychological morbidity in the [D-Trp[6]]LHRH group. All the patients were aware of the diagnosis of a malignant disease and this probably resulted in an equivalent degree of psychological stress in both groups and increased stress (expected from the orchiectomy group) was not detected in this study. Following orchiectomy a large proportion of patients were implanted with synthetic prostheses and this probably resulted in less psychological morbidity than was originally anticipated.

Although the response rates to orchiectomy and [D-Trp[6]]LHRH are equivalent there are a number of factors that should determine what is the best first line treatment for advanced prostatic cancer. Orchiectomy has the advantage of an immediate reduction in testosterone which later does not require continued administration of drug to suppress testosterone. It is not associated with any significant long term sequelae and is relatively cheap. The disadvantages include inpatient care for a few days in hospital and the usual anaesthetic risk. Further, a proportion of patients fail to respond to orchiectomy and have therefore been subjected to an operation that is unnecessary, potentially psychologically damaging and expensive in such patients. Psychological morbidity due to bilateral orchiectomy has not been clearly addressed previously, though it has always been deemed a major factor. Certainly psychological morbidity is significant in the presence of life-threatening disease and needs to be taken into account [27]. Our results indicate that the psychological morbidity with orchiectomy may be only slightly greater than in such patients treated by other means. The psychological impact of the cancer seems to override the immediate impact of the orchiectomy. However when patients are given a choice, at the start of treatment, which is now often demanded by some patients, a large proportion choose to have monthly injections rather than surgical orchiectomy. Indeed one can now argue that all patients with advanced prostatic cancer should be given LHRH agonists for three months and thereafter select those patients who have responded, for orchiectomy, which for this group of patients works out cheaper the longer the duration of remission is maintained.

The GnRH agonist has the advantage that it can be administered by intramuscular injection once a month, has no significant side-effects and compliance can be virtually guaranteed in an outpatient setting. In the present climate of increasing public awareness, patients may wish to make an active informed choice between the different treatments available for advanced prostatic cancer. Whilst some patients may choose orchiectomy others may prefer a simple injection every month. In view of this and since the costs of these drugs are likely to come down we have no hesitation in recommending long acting [D-Trp[6]]LHRH as a safe and highly effective alternative to orchiectomy for first line treatment of advanced prostatic cancer.

ACKNOWLEDGEMENTS

We would like to thank the following clinicians for contributing patients for the study: L. Allen, FRCS, Edgware General Hospital, Edgware; N. Singh, FRCS, Whipps Cross Hospital, London; R. Notley, FRCS, Royal Surrey County Hospital, Guildford; F. Schweitzer,

114

FRCS, Royal Surrey Hospital, Guildord; J. Towler, FRCS, Luton & Dunstable Hospital, Luton and J. Fleming, FRCS, West Middlesex Hospital, London.

REFERENCES

1.   Schally, AV, Coy, DH and Arimura, A (1980). LHRH agonists and antagonists. Int J Gynaecol Obstet, 18, 318
2.   Tolis, G, Ackman, D, Stellos, A, Mehta, A, Labrie, F, Fazekas, AT, Comaru-Schally, AM and Schally, AV (1982). Tumour growth inhibition in patients with prostatic carcinoma treated with luteinizing hormone-releasing hormone agonists. Proc Natl Acad Sci USA, 79, 1658
3.   Allen, JM, O'Shea, JP, Mashiter, K, Williams, G and Bloom, SR (1983). Advanced carcinoma of the prostate: treatment with a gonadotrophin releasing hormone agonist. Brit Med J, 286, 1607
4.   Walker, KJ, Turkes, AO, Nicholson, RI, Turkes, A and Griffiths, K (1983). Therapeutic potential of the LHRH agonist ICI 118630, in the treatment of advanced prostatic carcinoma. Lancet, 1, 413
5.   Waxman, JH, Wass, JAH, Hendry WF, Whitfield, HN, Besser, GM, Malpas, JS and Oliver, RTD (1983). Treatment with gonadotrophin releasing hormone analogue in advanced prostatic cancer. Brit Med J, 286, 1309
6.   Comite, F, Cutler, GB Jr, Rivier, J, Vale, WW, Loriaux, DL and Crowley, WF Jr (1981). Short term treatment of idiopathic precocious puberty with a long-acting analogue of LHRH: a preliminary report. N Engl J Med, 305, 1546
7.   Meldrum, DR, Chang, RJ, Lu, J, Vale, W, Rivier, J and Judd, HL (1982). "Medical oophorectomy" using a long acting GnRH agonist - a possible approach to the treatment of endometriosis. J Clin Endocrinol Metab, 54, 1081
8.   Parmar, H, Nicholl, J, Stockdale, A, Cassoni, A, Phillips, RH, Lightman, SL and Schally, AV (1985). Advanced ovarian carcinoma: Response to the agonist [D-Trp^6]LHRH. Cancer Treat Rep, 69, 1341
9.   Lorr, M, Daston, P and Smith, IR (1967). An analysis of mood states. Education and Psychological Measurement, 27, 89
10.   Johnston, M and Hackman, A (1977). Cross validation and response sets in repeated use of mood questionnaires. Brit J Soc Clin Psychol, 16, 235
11.   Melzack, R (1985). The McGill pain questionnaire. Major properties and scoring methods. Pain, 1, 277
12.   Huggins, C and Hodges, CV (1941). Studies on prostatic cancer. I. The effect of castration, of oestrogen and of androgen injection on serum phosphatases in metastatic carcinoma of the prostate. Cancer Res, 1, 293
13.   Huggins, C, Stevens, RE Jr and Hodges, CV (1941). Studies on prostatic cancer. II. The effects of castration on advanced carcinoma of the prostate gland. Arch Surg, 43, 209

14.   Byars, DP (1973). The veterans administration cooperative urological research group's studies of cancer of the prostate. Cancer, 32, 1126

15.   Kirk, D (1985). Prostatic cancer. Brit Med J, 290, 875

16.   Klugo, RC, Farah, RN and Cerny, JC (1981). Bilateral orchidectomy: response of serum testosterone and clinical response to subsequent oestrogen therapy. Urology, 17, 49

17.   Ferguson, JD (1975). Limits and indications for adrenalectomy and hypophysectomy in the treatment of prostatic cancer. In Braccu U, Di Silverio F (eds.). "Hormonal Therapy of Prostatic Cancer". p. 201. (Palermo: Cofese Edizioni)

18.   West, CW and Murphy, GP (1973). Pituitary ablation and disseminated prostatic carcinoma. JAMA, 225, 253

19.   Farnsworth, WE (1972). Prolactin and the prostate. In Boynes AR and Griffiths, K (eds.) "Prolactin and Carcinogenesis". p. 217. (Cardiff: Alpha omega Alpha)

20.   Altwein, JE and Jacobi, GH (1981). Adjunctive bromocriptine therapy in advanced prostatic cancer. Antihormone. In "Bedeutung in der Urologie". p. 223. (München: Zuckswherdt Verlag)

21.   Mee, AD, Khan, O and Mashiter, K (1984). High serum prolactin associated with poor prognosis in carcinoma of the prostate. Brit J Urol, 56, 698

22.   The Leuprolide Study Group (1984). Leuprolide versus diethylstilbestrol for metastatic prostate cancer. N Engl J Med, 311, 1281

23.   Ellis, WJ and Grayhack, JT (1963). Sexual function in aging males after orchidectomy and oestrogen therapy. J Urol, 89, 895

24.   Bergman, B, Damber, JE, Littbrand, B, Sjögren, K and Tomic R (1984). Sexual function in prostatic cancer patients treated with radiotherapy, orchiectomy or oestrogens. Brit J Urol, 56, 64

25.   Sogani, PC, Vagiawala, MR and Whitmore, WF (1984). Experience with flutamide in patients with advanced prostatic carcinoma without prior endocrine therapy. Cancer, 54, 744

26.   McGowan, DG (1977). Radiation therapy in the management of localized carcinoma of the prostate. A preliminary report. Cancer, 39, 98

27.   Anderson, BL (1985). Sexual functioning morbidity among cancer survivors. Cancer, 55, 1835

11

ORCHIDECTOMY VERSUS TOTAL ANDROGEN BLOCKADE. A PHASE III EORTC 30853 STUDY

L. DENIS, F. KEUPPENS, D. NEWLING, P.H. SMITH,
F. CALAIS DA SILVA, R. SYLVESTER, M. DE PAUW. P. ONEGANA and
Members of the EORTC GU Group, Belgium
A.Z. Middelheim, Antwerp 2020, Belgium

INTRODUCTION

The majority of patients with symptomatic prostatic cancer show objective and subjective responses when effective endocrine treatment blocks the androgen stimulation to the prostate. However, the correct choice of endocrine treatment is still an unanswered question.

Three consecutive prospective randomized phase III trials on more than 1000 patients (EORTC 30761, 30762, 30805) failed to identify superior treatment results by a variety of hormonal agents versus bilateral orchidectomy. The last treatment, usually in the form of the subcapsular removal of testicular tissue, removes the testicular source of androgens and is still considered as standard therapy forty years after its introduction to the treatment of advanced prostatic cancer [1].

Claims to better response rates in a phase II study by the simultaneous suppression of the testicular and the adrenal androgens led to the initiation of the presently described randomized phase III trial. The trial compares the therapeutic effect and safety of responses obtained after bilateral total or subcapsular orchidectomy versus a combination of a luteinizing hormone releasing hormone analogue (LHRH A) in a depot preparation together with the non steroidal anti-androgen, flutamide.

PATIENTS AND METHODS

Choice of treatment

The option of the participating centres as to the type of bilateral orchidectomy, total or subcapsular, was left open. There is a definitive trend towards the subcapsular removal of the endocrine testicular tissue for the obvious cosmetic and psychological results which favours a better acceptance by the patients. It has been demonstrated that the epididymis is able to produce androgenic steroids from the circulating adrenal C19 steroids or from cholesterol. This residual activity of androgenic stimulation is negligible in the clinical situation where the amounts of weaker adrenal androgens allow the prostatic tissue to sustain tissue levels of dihydrotestosterone (DHT) by peripheral metabolisation [2,3].

The combination treatment included the LHRH analogue ICI 118630 ([D-Ser(Bu^t)^6, Azgly^{10}]LHRH; Zoladex), and the non steroidal anti-androgen Schering 13521 (flutamide; 2-methyl-N-4-nitro-3 (trifluoromethyl)phenyl propamide; Eulexin).

The rationale for the Zoladex choice was based on our previous phase II study with the slow release (depot) formulation with the analogue incorporated in a 50:50 lactide:glycolide co-polymer in the form of a small injectable rod. Injection of a 3.6 mg dose every four weeks, corresponding to a daily release of 120 µg Zoladex/day, reduced plasma testosterone levels to castrate levels by the second week in all patients in this multicenter phase II trial [4]. No treatment superiority can be demonstrated versus other forms of LHRH analogues but the reliable monthly depot preparations improve patient compliance compared to pernasal or daily intramuscular preparations [5]. There were no serious side effects except for the possibility of an exacerbation of disease symptoms from the initial stimulation of a sudden rise in plasma testosterone (common to all LHRH agonists) and the endocrine reaction to a subsequent drop in plasma testosterone (hot flushes, lack of libido, impotence). The addition of diethylstilb- estrol, cyproterone acetate, ketoconazole or as in this trial, flutamide, in the first weeks of treatment completely eliminates the early exacerbation of symptoms [3,5].

The choice for flutamide in the combination treatment was based on the safety record in earlier studies with no reports of cardio-vascular toxicity [6]. Aside from infrequent nausea, diarrohea and transient elevations of liver enzymes, the most common adverse effects were gynaecomastia and breast tenderness.

TRIAL DESIGN

This open, randomised phase III trial was activated in March 1986 by the urological group of the European Organisation of Treatment and Research of Cancer (EORTC) under the code number 30853. The protocol was prepared by a group of urologists, endocrinologists, data managers and one statistician and after four revisions approved by the EORTC protocol review committee in December 1986.

One coordinator responsible for the overall organisation and liaison to the EORTC Data Center (L. Denis), one coordinator responsible for the comparative evaluation with the previous EORTC study 30805 (M. Robinson), one coordinator responsible for the endocrine aspects (C. Mahler) and a specially assigned data manager (P. Ongena) form the coordination committee of the trial.

Quality control was officially envigilated by different ad hoc committees on central pathology (P.J. Spaander), endocrine aspects (C. Mahler), bone scan evaluation (P.H. Smith), response criteria (D. Newling), quality of life (F. Calais da Silva) and research aspects (T. Cooper). The complete list of collaborators is given in Appendix 1.

The objectives of the trial were: 1) To compare the efficacy and safety of orchidectomy plus Zoladex and Flutamide in delaying progression of metastatic carcinoma of the prostate (M1 disease) and in prolonging survival in a prospective two arm randomized trial. 2) To determine the incidence and duration of responses for each treatment arm. The trial was designed to incorporate at least 226 patients based on the following statistical considerations: In order to detect a difference of 50% in the median time to progression between the 2 treatment arms, 96 patients followed until progression will be required in each arm (α - 0.05, β - 0.20); since 85% of the patients can be expected to progress during the course of follow-up (5 years), a total of approximately 226 evaluable patients will be required. Assuming an entry rate of 100 patients per year, the required number of patients will be entered in 2 to 3 years; 113 evaluable patients on each arm will also be sufficient to detect a difference of 20% in the response rate on the 2 arms (α - .50, β - .20). In our last quality control meeting on this trial it was decided, due to excellent accrual, to randomise up to 320 patients till May 1988.

All patients admitted to the participating clinical centres with histologically proven carcinoma of the prostate with M1 category disease according to the UICC 1978 TNM criteria [7] were eligible for entry to the study if they had a performance status of WHO 0-2 criteria with a life expectancy of at least three months. All, T, N and G categories were allowed. Bone metastases could be diagnosed by bone scan and/or any type of X rays but questionable metastases should be biopsied. A written informed consent according to local hospital regulations was required from all patients before randomisation. Patients who received previous hormonal or chemotherapy and those with concurrent malignancy except skin cancer were excluded from the trial. Other criteria for exclusion included age over 80, obvious lever pathology (twice normal values of the transaminases) and cooperative problems due to psychiatric disorders or too large a distance from the centre for adequate follow-up.

Following randomisation, patients remained with their assigned treatment group which was given, if possible, for a minimum of 3 months. Patients who responded or did not change followed treatment until progression. Upon progression patients went off treatment but were followed for survival. Clinical evaluation was done every 4 weeks for 3 months, then every 12 weeks for 48 weeks and thereafter every 24 weeks.

REGISTRATION AND RANDOMISATION OF PATIENTS

Patients were registered by a telephone call to the EORTC Data Center. The date of registration was the date of making the call. The basic registration data included the protocol number, the name and number of the institution, the name of the patient, the performance status and the names of the urologist and the local pathologist.

The on study form and the on study pathology form were sent within one month to the Data Center. A copy of the on study pathology form was sent to Central Pathology with three unstained slides of the initial histological material. Central Pathology confirmed the diagnosis and the grade and informed the local pathologist.

THERAPEUTIC REGIMEN

Bilateral orchidectomy was performed under local or general anesthesia. Zoladex depot 3.6 mg was given subcutaneously every four weeks till the patient went off study. The time between two injections was not to exceed 35 days to avoid normalisation of serum testosterone levels. Flutamide 250 mg three times a day was given in addition with 150 cc of water after meals.

PRETREATMENT STUDIES AND FOLLOW-UP

The initial studies included a general history which include all symptoms referable to prostatic cancer (e.g. performance status, pain and micturition problems). The scoring system for this information is presented in Appendix 2.

A special 33 point quality of life questionnaire prepared by the quality of life committee was optional. This questionnaire was repeated every month to improve patient compliance. A one time questionnaire was prepared to analyse the quality of life data from all patients on study with a minimum of 6 months follow-up. The physical examination included height, weight, blood pressure, presence of oedema, rectal examination where the two largest perpendicular measurements of the prostatic tumor were recorded, enlargement of lymph nodes and measurement of measurable lesions.

The measurements of the tumor by rectal examination were correlated in the study of the response criteria with the results obtained by transrectal ultrasound. The laboratory examinations include sedimentation rate, haemoglobin, hematocrit, gamma GT, transaminases and creatinine. White cell count and platelets were only taken in cases of anemia (Hb <7.8 nmol/P). Acid and akaline phosphatase as well as prostatic acid phosphatase were taken before or 48 hours after rectal examination. The prostatic acid phosphatase as well as the prostatic specific antigen and the acute phase proteins were part of the research side study on serological markers of prostatic cancer activity. The deep frozen samples taken at regular intervals were run centrally in the Unit for Cancer Research in Leeds. Participation in this study was optional.

The imaging examinations included a nuclear bone scan, X rays of hot spots on the bone scan, urography, liver ultrasound, chest X ray and ultrasound of the prostate (optional) or CT scan of the pelvis (optional).

The patient was seen at 4, 8 and 12 weeks after the start of treatment. He was then seen every 12 weeks for 48 weeks and thereafter every 24 weeks. At each visit the performance status, pain and micturition problems were recorded.

Patients in the quality of life studies were seen every four weeks to avoid time lapse bias between the two treatment arms. Some or all of the pretreatment examinations were repeated at regular intervals until the patient went off study. The study plan is presented in Table 1.

The patients went off study if: objective progression was documented; serious adverse reactions were experienced from the treatment, or the patient became unable or neglected to take his treatment. All patients were followed for progression and survival.

Objective proof of progression was the pivotal point of the study. Objective criteria for progression include: New hot spots on a bone scan which persists at a subsequent control scan one month later or are confirmed by X ray changes and/or proven at biopsy; new soft tissue lesions which are palpable and/or confirmed by CT scan and/or biopsy; new pulmonary or liver metastases. Increase in any measurable metastatic lesion by more than 25%. Note that increase in the intensity of hot spots or increase in size was not accepted as progression. Local progression was defined as an increase of >50% of the product of the two maximum perpendicular diameters of the primary tumor by rectal examination or by ultrasound scanning. Since very small changes in small volume glands would lead to the above criteria being fulfilled they would only be acceptable in patients whose tumor had at least one perpendicular diameter greater than 3cm. Transurethral resection of the primary lesion necessitated discontinuation of the use of the primary lesion as a parameter for progression. The patient was kept on study and evaluation of all other parameters continued, however.

Non specific and subjective criteria of progression included: increase of acid phosphatase (measured by biochemical or immunological methods) by 100% or more noted on two successive occasions, one month apart; changes in performance status – worsening of 2 scores; changes in pain and use of analgesics – worsening of 2 scores, or from 3 to 4; changes in urinary symptoms to 3; weight loss of 10% or greater. Subjective deterioration in a patient's general condition alone was not a valid reason to withdraw the patient from the study. Likewise an improvement of the performance after radio-therapy of metastatic lesions was not regarded as a criterion for response. Spontaneous fracture of bone was not evidence of progression. Other criteria of response included complete response, partial response and no change. All patients were followed till death.

Table 1. Study plan for patients with stage M1 prostatic cancer (two treatment arms)

Duration of Treatment	Before Treatment							During Treatment Period
Date	first year							after first year
weeks	0	4	8	12	24	36	48	every 24 weeks
visit	1	2	3	4	5	6	7	7 8
Informed consent	+							
Anamnesis (complaints, side effects, medication)	+	+	+	+	+	+	+	+
Physical examination	+	+	+	+	+	+	+	+
Laboratory	+			+	+	+	+	+
Hematology	+			+	+	+	+	+
Blood chemistry	+			+	+	+	+	+
Acid/alkaline phosphatase	+			+	+	+	+	+
General urinanalysis	+							
Endocrinology	+	+		+	+	+	+	at time of progression
Testosterone								every 48 weeks and at time of progression
Radiology								
Specific skeletal lesions	+				+	+		+
Bone scan	+				+	+		+
IVP							(+)	if indicate
CAT scan	(+)				(+)			(+)
Ultrasound of prostate	(+)				(+)			(+)
Chest x-ray	+					+		+
Ultrasound of liver	(+)							(+)
Histology primary tumour	+							
Cytology	(+)							(+)

(+) = optional

RESULTS AND DISCUSSION

Two hundred and fifty eight patients were randomized in the study between March 1986 and October 1987. Ten patients (4%) were ineligible mainly because of the age >80 years or randomisation errors. A total of 20 institutions entered 248 eligible patients as presented in Table 2. The patient characteristics were

Table 2. Patient entry by institution.

Institution	No. of Patients
A.Z. Middleheim-A.Z. Vub, Brussels	36
Santa Maria, Lisbon	28
Princess Royal, Hull	24
St. James, Leeds	22
Varese	18
Castleford	18
Leuven	16
Baviere, Liege	12
St. Jozef, Oostende	11
O.L.V., Aalst	10
York	9
Do Desterro, Lisbon	9
Strasbourg	9
Univ. St. Luc, Brussels	6
Freeman, Newcastle	6
A.Z. Gent	5
Palermo	4
St. Radboud, Nijmegen	3
Barmherzigen Bruder, Munchen	2

analysed for all subjective and objective criteria and found to be evenly distributed between the two treatment arms. The urological symptoms and the T category on rectal examination are presented in Tables 3 and 4.

Table 3. Zoladex and flutamide vs. bilateral orchidectomy: patient characteristics for symptoms.

Urological Symptoms	None	Moderate	Severe	Total
Bilateral Orchidectomy	8.2	23.2	16.4	47.8
Zoladex & flutamide	8.2	25.8	18.2	52.2
Total	16.4	49.0	34.6	100.0

TOTAL 159 IN %

Two hundred and nine patients (91.3%) out of 229 evaluable patients were still on study after 18 months. The number of patients that went off study for progression of disease was 13 (5.7%) of which 8 were in the orchidectomy arm while the remaining five were in the medical treatment arm.

Table 4. Zoladex and flutamide vs. bilateral orchidectomy patients characteristics for stage.

T Category	T0	T1	T2	T3	T4	Total
Bilateral Orchidectomy	0	4.4	8.8	23.1	11.2	47.5
Zoladex & Flutamide	1.2	5.6	11.2	19.4	15.0	52.5
Total	1.2	10.0	20.0	42.5	26.2	100.0

Preliminary results are available for 146 patients on endocrine side effects. These were mainly hot flashes and gynaecomastia and the incidence was not different between the two treatments.

Not one single case of adverse effect by the so called "flare up" phenomenon was reported. This confirms the reported prevention of peak levels of testosterone with aggravation of symptoms by the addition of flutamide to the LHRH agonist therapy [8].

In the side studies it was noted that up to 69% of the patients have a second measurement of the primary tumor after rectal evaluation by some type of imaging of the prostate. Transrectal ultrasound was the preferred control technology in 56% of the cases.

The side study on bone scan revealed that 26% of the evaluated 161 patients had hot spots and negative X rays while 70% had both hot spots and positive X rays .

The bone scan committee recommended comparison of the incidences of remission on the bone scan to other criteria of response, to establish the necessity of the bone scan as a follow up evaluation. The results of the side study proved so important that it was moved from optional to obligatory in the treatment evaluation. It is far too early to evaluate the results of the analysis for markers, especially prostatic specific antigen (PSA). From our personal patients in the study we expect to find confirmation of the PSA determination as a sensitive indicator of response to treatment [9].

This study will be closed in May 1988 with the expected accrual number of 320 patients. This preliminary report shows no statistical difference in time to progression between the two treatment arms. We hope that the inbuilt quality control by the side studies will allow a clear evaluation of the different subjective and objective criteria utilised in this study. The comparison between the different parameters will be made on a semi-blind basis with assessments of responses to treatment made in isolation of the assessments of the endpoints of the study. We hope that the results of this study will improve on the monitoring of established paramaters in future studies on advanced prostatic cancer and that we will receive a straightforward answer on the efficacy and safety from both treatments.

REFERENCES

1.   Parmar, H, Edwards, L, Phillips, RH, Allen, L and Lightman, SL (1987). Orchiectomy versus long-acting D-Trp-6-LHRH in advanced prostatic cancer. Brit J Urol, 59, 248
2.   Senge, T, Hulshoff, T, Tunn, U, Schenck, B and Neumann, F (1978). Testosteronkonzentratien in serum nach subkapsularer orchidektomie. Urologe A, 177, 382
3.   Labrie, F, Dupont, A and Belanger, A (1985). Complete androgen blockade for the treatment of prostate cancer. In: DeVita, VT Jr, Hellman, S and Rosenberg, SA (eds.). "Important Advances in Oncology 1985". p.193. (Philadelphia: JB Lippincott Company)
4.   Denis, L, Keuppens, F, Mahler, C, Debruyne, FMJ, Weil, EHJ, Lunglmayr, G, Newling, D, Robinson, MRG, Richards, B, Smith, PH and Whelman, P (1987). Long term therapy with a depot LHRH analogue (Zoladex R) in patients with advanced prostatic cancer. In: Murphy, GP, Khoury, S, Küss, R, Chatelain, R and Denis, L (eds.) "Prostate Cancer Part A: Research, Endocrine Treatment, and Histopathology". p.221. (New York: AR Liss Inc.)
5.   Denis, L (1988). Luteinizing hormone releasing hormone agonists. In: Denis, L (ed.) "Medical Management of Prostatic Cancer". p.49. (Berlin: Springer Verlag)
6.   Prout, G, Griffin, P, Keating and Schiff (1988). Long-term experience with Flutamide in patients with prostatic carcinoma. J Urol (in press)
7.   Harmer, MH (1987). TNM Classification of Malignant Tumours. 3rd Edition (Geneva: International Union Against Cancer)
8.   Denis, L and Mahler, C (1988). LHRH agonists combination studies . In: Motta, M and Serio, M (eds.) "Hormonal Therapy of Prostatic Diseases: Basic and Clinical Aspects". (In press) (Apeldoorn: Medicom Europe BV)
9.   Siddall, JK, Hetherington, JW, Cooper, EH, Newling, DWW, Robinson, MRG, Richards, B and Denis L (1986). Biochemical monitoring of carcinoma of prostate treated with an LH-RH analogue (Zoladex). Brit J Urol, 58, 676

Appendix 1. Collaborators EORTC 30853.

Zoladex and Flutamide Vs. Bilateral Orchidectomy

Protocol Authors:

D. Newling, P. Smith, M. Robinson, B. Richards (UK)
F. DeBruyne, H. De Voogt, J. Klign, F. Schroder (NL)
F. Calais Da Silva (P)
A. Bono (I)
G. Lunglmayr (A)
S. Fossa (N)
C. Bouffioux, L. Denis, F. Keuppens, C. Mahler (B)

Coordination Committee:

Study Coordinator	: L. Denis (B)
Co-Coordinators	: M. Robinson (UK)
	C. Mahler (B)
Study Data Manager	: P. Ongena (B)

Data Center:

Statistician	: R. Sylvester (US)
Data Managers	: M. De Pauw (B)
	B. Hammond (B)

Initiated March 1986
Closed   May   1988

Appendix 2. Scoring system for EORTC 30853

1. <u>WHO Performance Status</u>:

   0   Able to carry out all normal activity without restriction

   1   Restricted in physically strenuous activity but ambulatory and able to carry out light work

   2   Ambulatory and capable of all self-care but unable to carry out any work, up and about more than 50% of waking hours

   3   Capable of only limited self-care, Confined to bed or chair more than 50% of waking hours

   4   Completely disabled, cannot carry on self-care, totally confined to bed or chair

2. <u>Pain</u>:

   0   No pain

   1   Mild (non-narcotic analgesics occasionally required)

   2   Moderate (non-narcotic analgesics regularly required)

   3   Severe (narcotic analgesics occasionally required)

   4   Intractable (narcotic analgesics regularly required)

3. <u>Urological Symptoms</u>:

   0   No symptoms

   1   Minimal symptoms requiring no therapy

   2   Moderate symptoms requiring medical therapy

   3   Severe symptoms requiring surgical relief or catheterisation

12

TOWARDS THE BEST TREATMENT FOR ADVANCED PROSTATIC CANCER

Jonathan WAXMAN, Jurgen SANDOW, P. ABEL, N. FARAH,
J. FLEMING, J. COX, E.P.N. O'DONOGHUE, K. SIKORA
and G. WILLIAMS
Department of Clinical Oncology, Hammersmith Hospital,
Du Cane Road, London W12 0HS, UK

INTRODUCTION

Gonadotrophin releasing hormone agonists have recently been introduced as an alternate medical treatment for prostatic cancer [1]. These compounds are without the cardiovascular toxicities of oestrogen therapy and obviate the need for orchiectomy. The agonists are initially stimulatory to the pituitary gonadal axis and as a result up to 40% of patients may have an acute exacerbation of the symptoms and signs of their malignancy. this may take the form of an increase in bone pain or lymphoedema, or more seriously cause obstructive uropathy or cord compression [2]. In this study, we have investigated ways of abrogating tumour flare comparing three different anti-androgen regimens given to patients about to receive gonadotrophin releasing hormone agonist therapy.

Current methods of applying gonadotrophin releasing hormone agonists are sub-optimal. It is inappropriate to treat elderly patients with five or six times daily nasal sprays or daily injection therapy. Recently, long-acting depot preparations of gonadotrophin releasing hormone agonists have become available [3]. Through modification of the co-polymer base, the release characteristics of these depot preparations can be altered. We have evaluated a new long-acting preparation of buserelin which is effective in suppressing testosterone in non-human primates for at least two months.

PATIENTS METHODS AND TREATMENT

PATIENTS

Thirty patients with symptomatic, locally advanced or metastatic disease gave informed consent to be treated in this study.

METHODS

All patients were staged according to the TNM classification of the UICC by physical examination, haemotological and biochemical

assessment, plain X-ray of the chest and pelvis and technitium
bone scan. Serum concentrations of acid and alkaline
phosphatases, testosterone, luteinizing hormone (LH) and follicle
stimulating hormone (FSH) were measured between 8.30 and 9.30 am
prior to treatment and on days 7, 8, 9, 10, 14, 21, 28 and 35 of
treatment. Thereafter, phosphatases, gonadotrophins and
testosterone were assessed weekly for the first six months of
treatment and subsequently monthly. Serum testosterone was
measured by radioimmunoassay after ether extraction.
Concentrations of LH and FSH were measured by specific double
antibody radio immunoassay, using MRC standards 68/40 and 78/549.

TREATMENT

Each patient was randomized to receive either 50mgs or 100mgs of
cyproterone acetate or Flutamide 250mgs thrice daily (tds) for one
week prior to and for the first month of buserelin therapy. After
7 days treatment with anti-androgen, each patient received 3.3mgs
of buserelin given in 75:25 lactide-glycolide co-polymer
formulation by subcutaneous implantation into the anterior
abdominal wall. At day 35, treatment with anit-androgen was

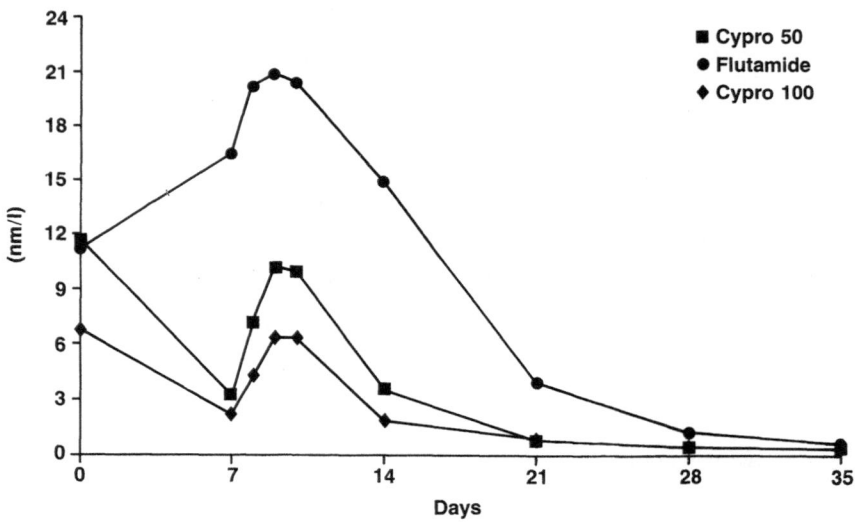

FIGURE 1 Effect of different adjunctive treatments on the serum
testosterone levels in patients treated with buserelin

discontinued and each patient received 6.6mgs of buserelin by
subcutaneous implantation at two monthly intervals.

RESULTS

1. Tumour flare.

(a) Cyproterone acetate 50mgs tds regimen:

Eight of this group of 10 patients had metastatic disease.
In 3 patients, there was an increase in bone pain occurring
between the third and seventh treatment days, which required in
one, opiate analgesia to control. A further patient within this
group developed renal failure, with serum creatinine increasing
from 133 nmol/l to 450 nmol/l at the third treatment week and then
resolving. This occurred in the context of a urinary tract
infection secondary to outflow obstruction.

(b) Cyproterone acetate 100mgs tds regimen:

Eight of 10 patients had metastatic disease. None of these
patients developed tumour flare during treatment.

(c) Flutamide 250mgs tds regimen:

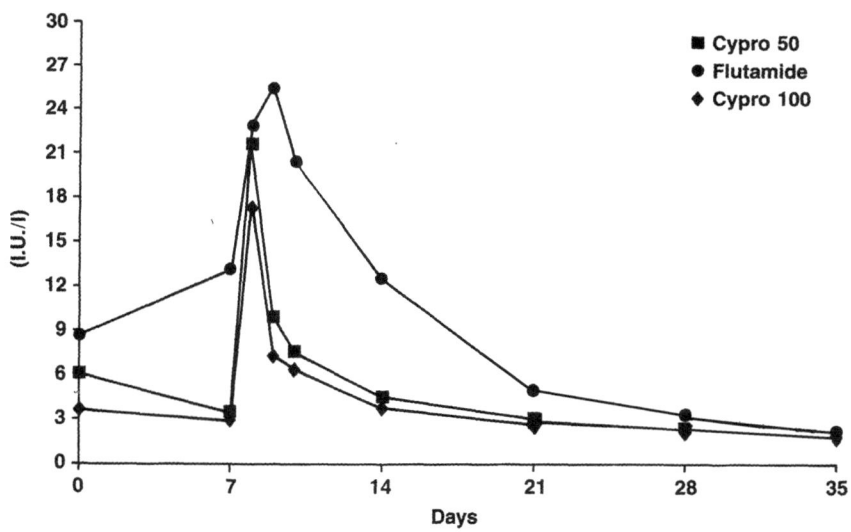

FIGURE 2 Effect of different adjunctive treatments on the
serum LH responses in patients treated with buserelin

Table 1: Changes in serum testosterone with treatment

(1) Cyproterone acetate 50 mg tds

Days	Mean	Testosterone (nmol/l) 95% confidence limits
0	11.7	7.7 – 17.7
7	3.2	2.0 – 5.0
8	7.2	4.4 – 11.7
9	10.2	6.0 – 17.0
10	10.0	5.9 – 16.5
14	3.5	2.4 – 4.9
21	0.7	0.5 – 1.1
28	0.4	0.3 – 0.6
35	0.3	0.3 – 0.4

(2) Cyproterone acetate 100 mgs tds

0	6.8	2.3 – 19.8
7	2.1	1.4 – 3.2
8	4.2	1.9 – 8.9
9	6.3	2.9 – 13.4
10	6.3	3.4 – 11.4
14	1.8	1.1 – 2.7
21	0.8	0.5 – 1.1
28	0.4	0.2 – 0.6
35	0.4	0.3 – 0.4

(3) Flutamide

0	11.1	6.7 – 18.2
7	16.4	9.6 – 27.9
8	20.2	11.5 – 35.3
9	20.9	11.7 – 37.3
10	20.4	11.4 – 36.7
14	14.9	8.1 – 27.4
21	3.9	2.1 – 7.4
28	1.2	0.7 – 1.9
35	0.6	0.0 – 0.0

Table 2:   Changes in LH with treatment

(1)   Cyproterone acetate 50 mg tds

Days	Mean	LH (IU/1) 95% confidence limits
0	6.1	4.6 – 8.0
7	3.4	2.4 – 4.6
8	21.5	16.4 – 28.2
9	10.0	7.1 – 13.8
10	7.5	5.8 – 9.6
14	4.5	3.7 – 5.2
21	3.0	2.5 – 3.6
28	2.5	2.0 – 3.2
35	2.3	1.7 – 3.0

(2)   Cyproterone acetate 100 mgs tds

Days	Mean	LH (IU/1) 95% confidence limits
0	6.8	3.7 – 12.8
7	4.3	2.8 – 6.5
8	28.0	17.5 – 44.9
9	10.4	7.3 – 14.9
10	8.9	6.4 – 12.2
14	5.2	3.8 – 7.1
21	3.8	2.6 – 5.4
28	3.3	2.3 – 4.6
35	2.5	1.8 – 3.5

(3)   Flutamide 250 mg tds

Days	Mean	LH (IU/1) 95% confidence limits
0	8.7	5.2 – 14.3
7	13.1	8.8 – 19.3
8	22.9	9.4 – 55.6
9	25.6	18.0 – 36.2
10	20.4	13.8 – 30.0
14	12.5	8.6 – 18.2
21	5.0	3.5 – 7.2
28	3.4	2.1 – 5.5
35	2.1	0.8 – 1.7

Table 3:   Changes in FSH with treatment

(1)   Cyproterone acetate 50 mg tds

Days	Mean	LH (IU/1) 95% confidence limits
0	4.1	2.8 - 5.7
7	1.7	1.2 - 2.4
8	8.3	5.8 - 11.8
9	4.7	3.1 - 6.8
10	3.2	2.1 - 4.6
14	1.5	1.2 - 1.8
21	1.1	1.0 - 1.2
28	1.2	1.0 - 1.4
35	1.3	1.0 - 1.6

(2)   Cyproterone acetate 100 mg tds

0	5.7	2.5 - 12.7
7	1.5	0.8 - 2.4
8	7.5	4.6 - 12.3
9	4.1	2.5 - 6.5
10	2.1	1.1 - 3.7
14	1.4	0.8 - 2.2
21	0.8	0.5 - 1.2
28	0.9	0.5 - 1.3
35	0.9	0.5 - 1.6

(3)   Flutamide 250 mg tds

0	4.6	2.8 - 7.4
7	6.2	4.0 - 9.5
8	8.9	5.9 - 13.2
9	5.7	3.5 - 9.2
10	5.2	3.2 - 8.1
14	2.3	1.4 - 3.5
21	1.2	0.9 - 1.5
28	1.3	1.0 - 1.5
35	1.1	1.0 - 1.2

Eight of this group of 10 patients had metastatic disease on presentation. In one patient, bone pain increased so that his oral opiate dosage had to be doubled to 200mgs tds of morphine slow release on the third day post-implantation. His pain began to resolve on the seventh post-implantation day.

2. Serum Gonadotrophins and Testosterone

Changes in mean serum concentrations of testosterone, LH and FSH in the first 35 days of treatment, are graphically represented in Figures 1, 2 and 3. Changes of serum testosterone, LH and FSH are

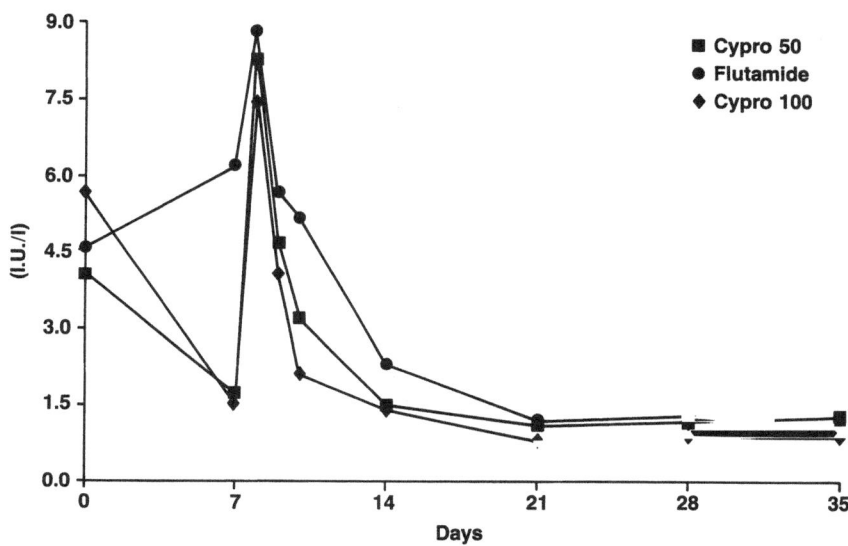

FIGURE 3 Effect of different adjunctive treatments on the serum FSH responses in patients treated with buserelin

detailed in Tables 1, 2 and 3. Log transformed data were analysed by one way analysis of variance in order to compare the changes in serum hormone levels within each of the patient groups. Peak serum testosterone levels were reached at Day 9 of treatment. Contrasting serum testosterone measurements at day 0 with day 9, Flutamide caused a significant increase in serum testosterone above base line, whereas the two cyproterone acetate regimens did not. The differences between the two cyproterone acetate regimens and Flutamide were significant (P=0.003). Contrasting day 7 with day 9, Flutamide as compared with both cyproterone acetate treated groups caused a significant increase in serum testosterone (P=0.004). There was no significant difference in peak levels of serum testosterone between the two groups of patients treated with different dosages of cyproterone acetate.

The difference between the groups in time to suppression of serum testosterone to the castrate range of less than 2.5 nmols/l was analysed by the Kruskal-Wallis test. The median number of

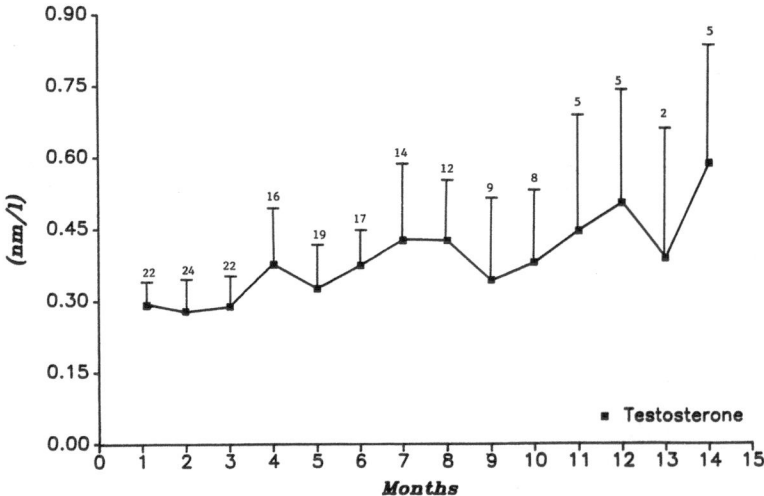

FIGURE 4 Serum testosterone levels in patients implanted with
6.6mg buserelin depot at 2 monthly intervals

days by which castrate levels of serum testosterone were obtained
was 14 days for the cyproterone acetate 100mgs tds regimen and 21
days for the cyproterone acetate 50mgs tds and Flutamide treated
patients. This difference was significant (P=0.001). Changes in
serum testosterone over the duration of treatment are detailed in
Figure 4. Testosterone remained in the castrate range in all
patients, treated for up to 14 months.

There was no significant increase in serum LH when
pre-treatment levels were compared to peak levels reached at day
8. However, comparing day 7 with day 8, LH increased significantly in the Flutamide treated patients as compared with both
groups of cyproterone acetate treated patients (P=0.001).
Comparing days 0 and 35, there was no significant change in LH in
any treated group.

Contrasting FSH levels in both group, peak levels were
achieved at day 8 and were significantly higher, (P<0.001), in the
Flutamide treated patients, as compared to both groups of cyproterone acetate treated patients. Comparing day 0 and day 35,
levels of FSH in all groups of patients were not significantly
suppressed.

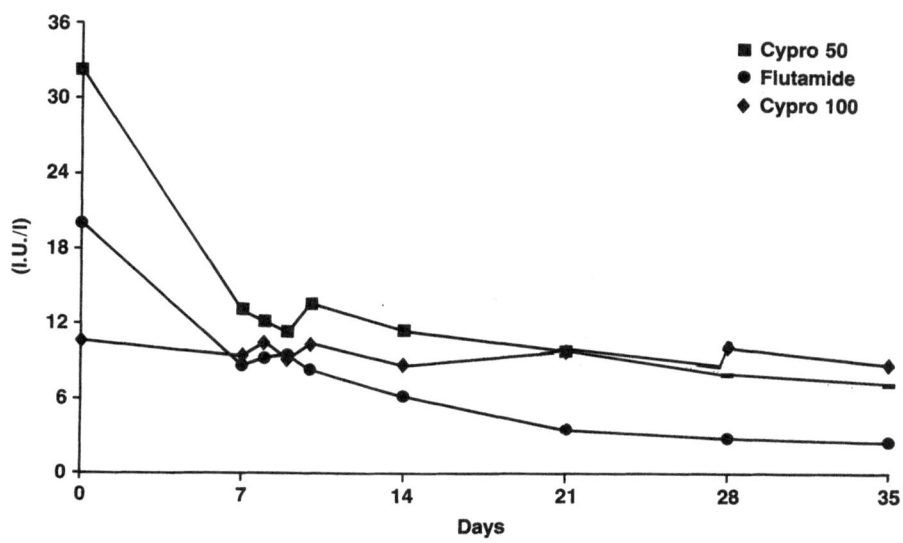

FIGURE 5 Effect of different adjunctive treatments on serum acid
phosphatase levels in patients treated with buserelin

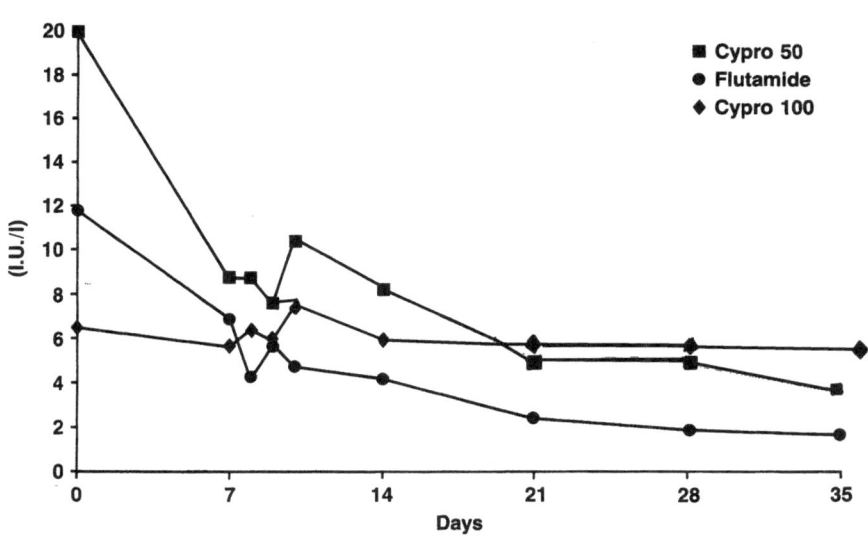

FIGURE 6 Effect of different adjunctive treatments on serum
prostatic acid phosphatase levels in patients treated with
buserelin

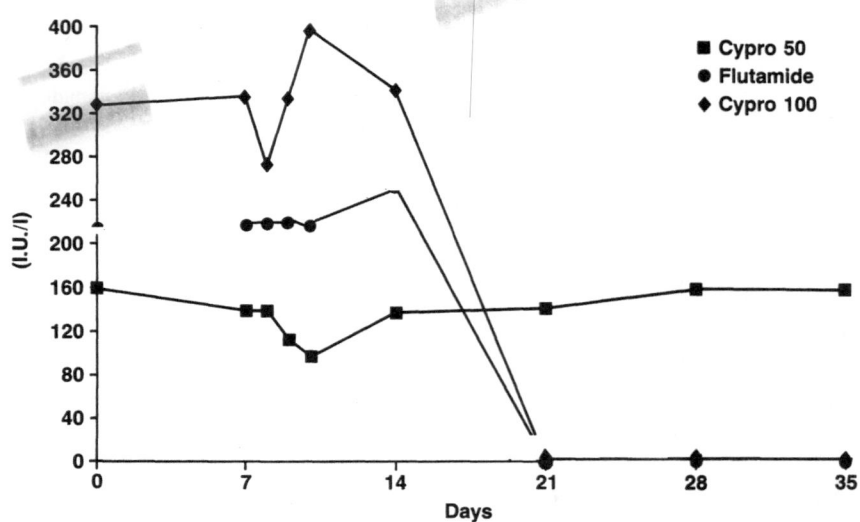

FIGURE 7   Effect of different adjunctive treatments on serum
           alkaline phosphatase levels in patients treated with buserelin

3. Serum phosphatases

Changes in serum concentrations of the phosphatases are described
in Figures 5, 6 and 7.   During the first month of treatment there
were no significant changes in serum levels of prostatic acid
phosphatase or alkaline phosphatase.   However, total acid
phosphatase increased significantly in the cyproterone acetate 100
mgs tds treated patients (P=0.04).   This increase was maximal at
the tenth treatment day.

4. Buserelin levels

Mean serum and urinary buserelin concentrations were measured
concomittantly with serum hormone and phosphatases levels during
the first month of treatment.   Subsequently, levels were measured
prior to implantation, at four hours post implantation and
thereafter weekly.

DISCUSSION

An endocrine and clinical evaluation has been performed of three
different anti-androgen regimens randomly applied to prevent
tumour flare in patients treated with buserelin.   In addition a
very long acting depot formulation of this agent has been

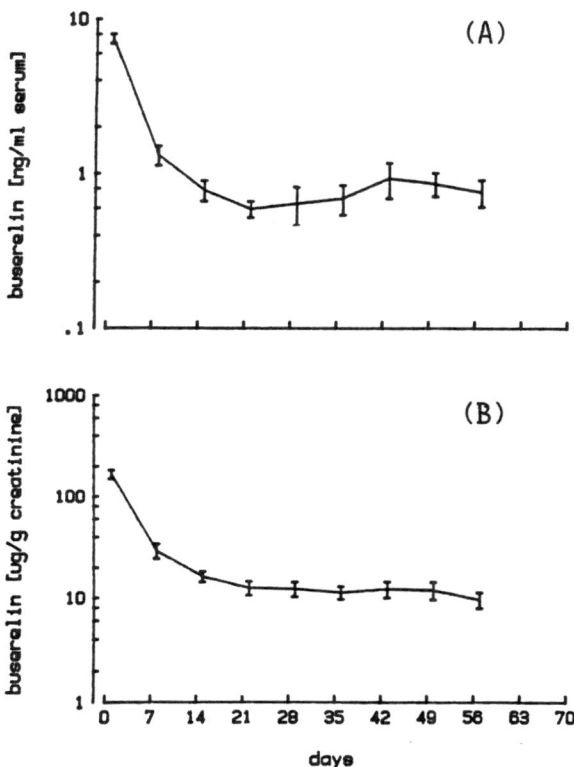

FIGURE 8   Serum (A) and urinary (B) levels of buserelin in
    patients implanted at 8 week intervals with 6.6mg of depot
    buserelin

pharmacologically assessed. Of the three anti-androgen regimens
given thrice daily for one week prior to treatment with depot
buserelin and for the first treatment month, cyproterone acetate
100mgs led to more rapid suppression of serum testosterone than
Flutamide 250mgs or cyproterone acetate 50mgs. There was a marked
difference in clinical efficacy. Cyproterone acetate 100mgs
thrice daily prevented tumour flare, a phenomenon that was seen
with both the lower dosage cyproterone acetate regimen and with
Flutamide. In all patients serum testosterone was maintained in
the castrate range for the duration of treatment which lasted up
to 14 months. This new depot preparation of buserelin should
therefore be considered as a step forward in the management of
patients with prostatic cancer.

We are now able to offer our patients minimally interven-
tional and safer treatment for prostatic cancer. The agonists
given in depot formulation every two months are effective in the
long-term suppression of serum testosterone. If cyproterone
acetate is given at 100mgs thrice daily for seven days prior to
and for the first month of treatment, tumour flare appears to be
prevented.

ACKNOWLEDGEMENTS

We thank Renate Biruls who complied the data, Mr. V. Aber who
performed the statistical analysis and Claire Wilson who typed the
manuscript.

REFERENCES

1.   Tolis, G, Ackman, D, Stellos, A, Metha, A, Labrie, F,
Fazekas AT and Comaru-Schally, AV (1982). Tumour growth inhibition in patients with prostatic carcinoma treated with luteinizing
hormone releasing-hormone agonists. Proc Natl Acad Sci USA, 79,
1658
2.   Waxman, JH, Man, A, Hendry, WF, Whitfield, HN, Besser, GM,
Tiptaft, RC, Paris, AM and Oliver, RTD (1985). Importance of
early tumour exacerbation in patients treated with long acting
analogues of gonadotrophin releasing hormone for advanced
prostatic cancer. Brit Med J, 291, 1387
3.   Waxman, JH, Sandow, J, Man, A, Barnett, MJ and Magill, PJ
(1986). The first clinical use of depot buserelin for advanced
prostatic carcinoma. Cancer Chemother Pharmacol, 18, 174

13

CLINICAL STUDIES OF LEUPROLIDE DEPOT FORMULATION IN METASTATIC PROSTATIC CANCER

Linda J. SWANSON, John H. SEELY, Robert BROWNELLER
and Devorah T. MAX
Abbott Laboratories, Abbott Park, IL 60064, USA

INTRODUCTION

Since the initial observation in 1976 that a GnRH analog, leuprolide, could be used to treat hormone-dependent tumors [1], many of these analogs have been synthesized and subsequently tested in the treatment of prostatic cancer and other hormone-dependent diseases. The first analogs to be studied were administered as daily subcutaneous injections. Later, formulations for intranasal administration were developed. Within the last few years, slow-release, long acting, depot formulations of some of these analogs have been produced and tested in man [2-4].

Lupron® (leuprolide acetate; TAP Pharmaceuticals), 1mg daily, is currently marketed as a daily subcutaneous injection for the palliative treatment of prostatic cancer. A 7.5 mg depot formulation of leuprolide acetate designed to release drug over a one month period was developed. Two studies have been conducted using this formulation:

METHODS

Study I

Fifty-three, previously untreated, stage D_2 prostatic cancer patients were evaluated in an open, multicenter study. The objective was to determine whether the leuprolide depot formulation injected once per month would reduce testosterone to castrate levels and maintain them within that range for the 6 months of treatment. The study was conducted in 10 centers in the United States beginning in March, 1986.

During this study all patients were treated with an intramuscular injection of 7.5 mg leuprolide as depot formulation at 28 day intervals. Testosterone (T), luteinizing hormone (LH), and leuprolide levels were determined one, or twice per week. The objective response to treatment, based on NPCP criteria, was assessed every 12 weeks. Patients remained in the study for as long as testosterone levels remained within the castrate range, and for as long as clinical benefit continued.

Fifty-six patients enrolled in the study, of whom 53 were evaluable for efficacy. The age range for patients enrolled in this study was 50-93 years; mean age was 68.2 ± 1 (S.E.M.) years. All patients had Stage D_2 disease and none had been previously treated. Patients enrolled in the study fulfilled the following entrance criteria: histologically confirmed prostatic adenocarcinoma in stage D_2 with two or more measurable or evaluable manifestations of prostatic cancer e.g., metastases, nodules in the prostate, or elevated serum acid phosphatase levels; testosterone levels of 150 ng/dl or more; performance status no greater than 2 (Eastern Cooperative Oncology Group Scale: ambulatory for more than 50% of waking hours, unless incapacitated by bone pain); no previous anticancer medication; recovery from the effects of major surgery. Radiation therapy to a metastatic site not used to determine response in this study, and provided two evaluable lesions remained, was permitted. Patients were excluded from the study if they had had orchiectomy, adrenalectomy or hypophysectomy and/or if they had a life prognosis of less than three months. All patients were required to sign an informed consent form.

Study II

The pharmacokinetic study was an open, single dose, study in 10 prostatic cancer patients who had been orchiectomized. Leuprolide measurements were made prior to the administration of the depot and at frequent intervals until Week 8. Leuprolide levels were determined in six patients beyond Week 8. Patients were included in the study who had had an orchiectomy at least one month prior to study entry and who had recovered from major surgery. Patients who had been treated with anticancer medication within four weeks preceding study entry, or who had a life prognosis of less than three months, were excluded from the study. All patients were required to sign an informed consent form.

RESULTS AND DISCUSSION

Testosterone Levels

The mean baseline T value prior to treatment was 370.6 ng/dl for the 53 evaluable patients (Fig. 1). There was an initial increase in mean serum T levels, with a peak at 552.7ng/dl on Day 4, after which levels fell, to well within the castrate range. Mean T levels had fallen to 33.8 ng/dl by Week 3, to 17.0 ng/dl by Week 4, and then remained less than 15 ng/dl through Week 24 of treatment.

The pattern of changes in serum LH over the 24 weeks was similar to that observed for testosterone (Fig. 2).

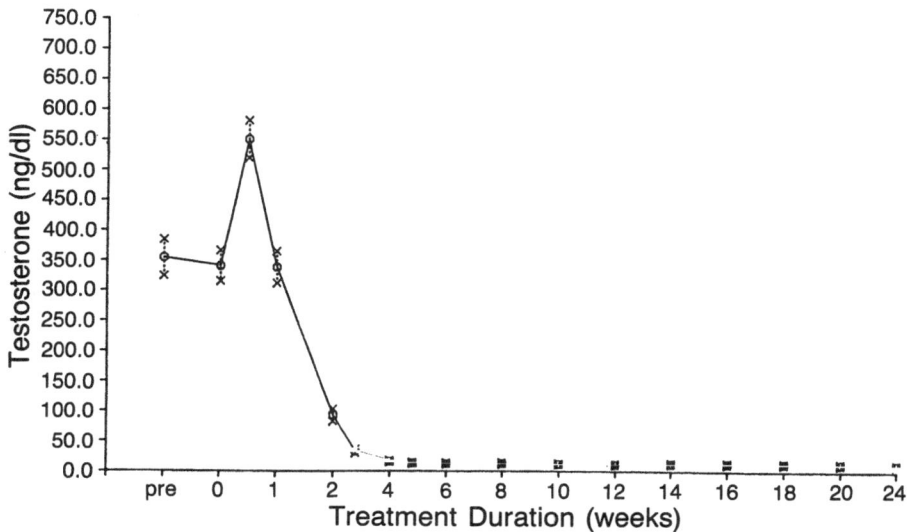

FIGURE 1 Mean (± S.E.M.) testosterone levels (ng/dl) over 24
weeks of therapy in previously untreated prostatic cancer
patients in Study I

Testosterone levels from 5 patients whose injections were
delayed by 7-12 days were considered to be non-evaluable until
injections were resumed on a regular basis, and T levels had once
again stabilized within the castrate range. Once injections had
resumed on a regular basis, the data could then be used in the
analysis of T levels. In the majority of cases a delay of the
injection by up to 12 days did not result in a clinically
significant increase in T levels. However, if an injection was
delayed by two or more weeks, T levels increased significantly.
        The first of two consecutive visits at which T levels were
≤50 ng/dl was considered as the "onset" of castrate levels of T.
The median time to onset of castrate testosterone levels for the
evaluable patients was 21 days. No patient showed an escape (two
consecutive tests at which T values were >50 ng/dl) from
suppression for the duration of their follow-up.
        Testosterone levels during this study were comparable to
those observed [6] with daily subcutaneous injection (30 mg/month)
of leuprolide (Fig. 3). The two dosage regimens were not
different in their ability to suppress serum T to castrate levels.

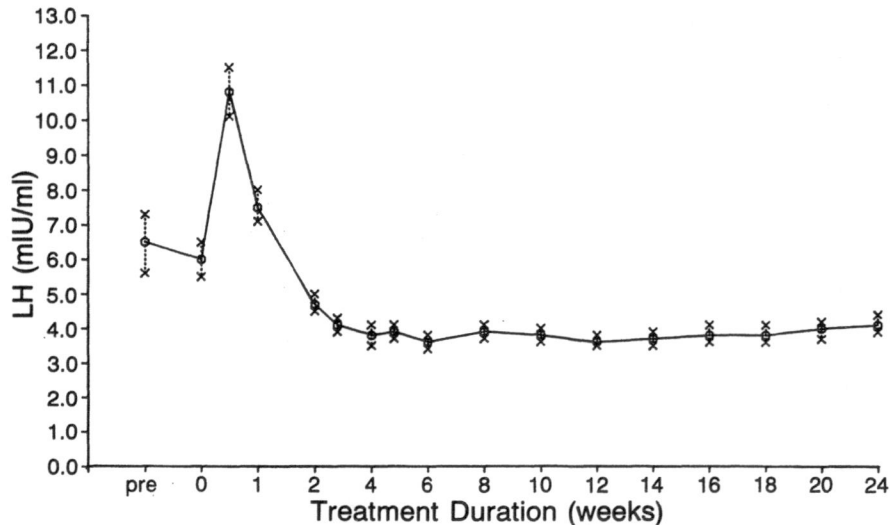

FIGURE 2   Mean (± S.E.M.) LH levels (mIU/ml) over 24 weeks of
    therapy in previously untreated prostatic cancer patients in
    Study I

Objective Tumor Response

Objective response to treatment was evaluated according to NPCP
criteria [5]. The best objective response observed for the 53
evaluable patients during 24 weeks of treatment is shown in
Table 1. Of the evaluable patients 1 was evaluated as a complete
responder (CR), 12 as partial responders (PR), and 30 as
objectively stable (NC) for a total no progression (CR + PR + NC)
rate of 81%. These responses are not statistically different from
those observed in the previous study in which prostate cancer
patients were treated with 1mg daily leuprolide injections [6].

Table 1 Best objective response Study I (i.m. depot injection) versus NDA study (leuprolide 1 mg/day subcutaneously) (minimum of 12 weeks therapy).

| Study | No Progression | | | | Progression | Total |
	CR	PR	NC	Total	P	Evaluated
I	1 (2%)	12 (23%)	30 (57%)	42 (81%)	10 (19%)	53 (100%)
NDA	1 (1%)	34 (37%)	44 (48%)	79 (86%)	13 (14%)	92 (100%)

CR = complete response. PR = partial response. NC = no change (objectively stable). P = progression.

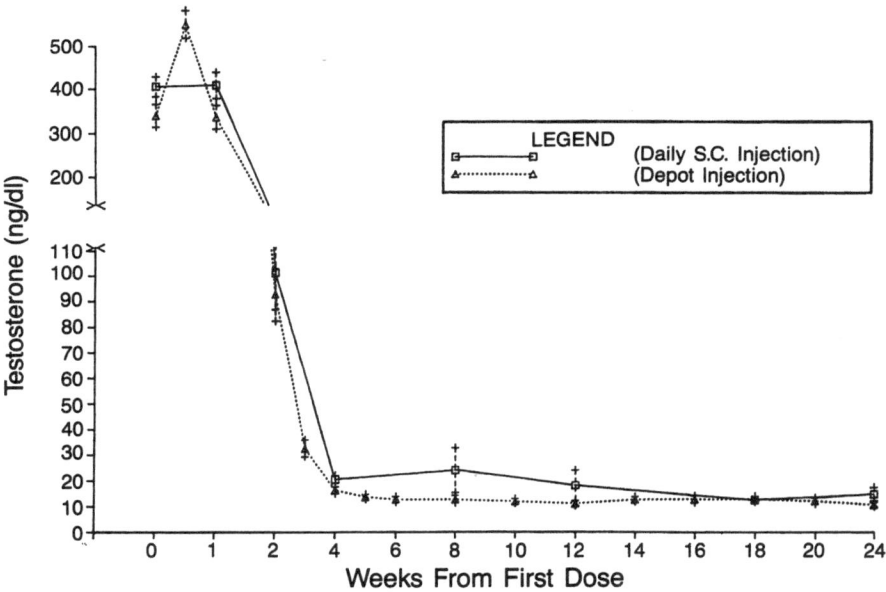

FIGURE 3 Comparison of mean (± S.E.M.) testosterone levels in previously untreated prostatic cancer patients over the first 24 weeks of treatment in Study I (leuprolide depot injection, 7.5 mg) and a previous [6] NDA Study, (1mg daily subcutaneous injection)

Leuprolide Levels

The depot injections were administered every 28 days, but the precise duration of drug release was not known. Thus, the possibility of an accumulation of leuprolide in the blood existed. However, the results indicated that there was no accumulation of plasma leuprolide during the 24 weeks of study (Fig. 4). Although, occasionally, leuprolide values were less than the limit of the assay sensitivity during the study, there was no corresponding increase in T levels after onset of castrate levels of T had occurred.

Study II

Pharmacokinetics

After an initial burst of leuprolide acetate in the plasma (which is characteristic of this type of dosage form) the levels declined to approximately 0.8ng/ml within 4 days after the injection, where they remained relatively stable for approximately 2.5 weeks (Fig. 5). By 4 weeks post-injection all patients but one still had measurable plasma levels of leuprolide. Drug levels continued to decline resulting in undetectable plasma levels, in the majority of patients, by 8 weeks post-injection.

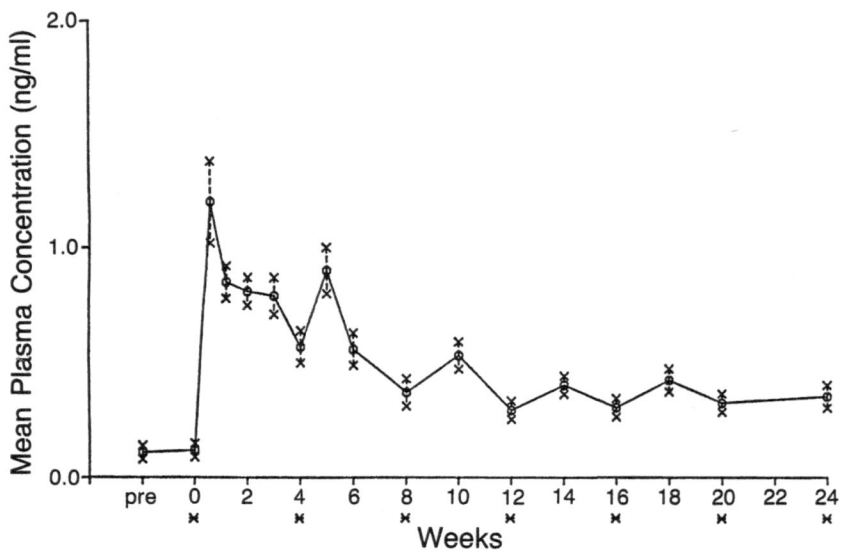

FIGURE 4 Mean (± S.E.M.) plasma leuprolide acetate concentrations (ng/ml) at each visit over 24 weeks of treatment in Study I (* = scheduled injection day).

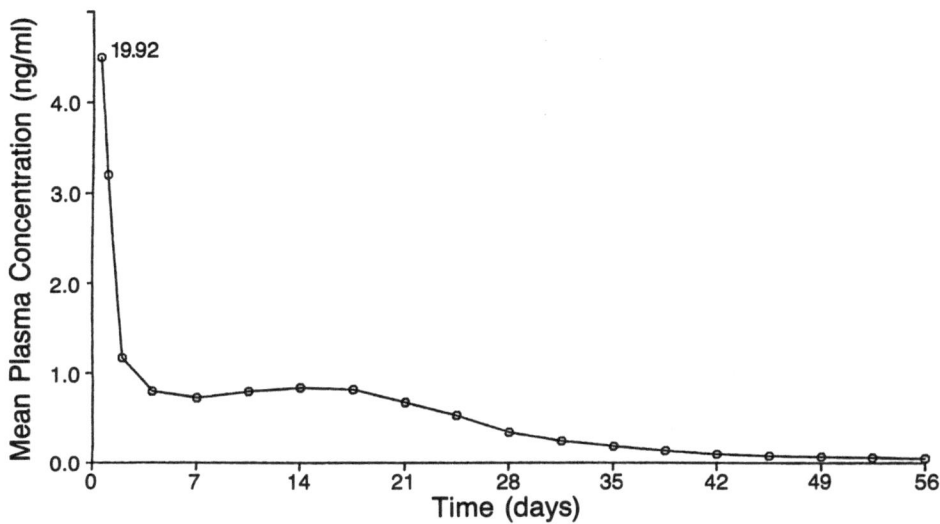

FIGURE 5   Mean plasma leuprolide acetate levels ng/ml) over 8
weeks following an intramuscular injection of the 7.5mg depot
in study II

Studies I and II

Adverse Events

All 66 patients 'from both studies were evaluated for adverse
events. Forty-five of the 56 patients who received leuprolide on
a monthly basis experienced one or more adverse events during the
first 24 weeks of treatment. The most common symptom was hot
flashes, which occurred in 32 patients. Sweating occurred in 6
patients, all of whom also experienced hot flashes. Events which
occurred in 5% or more of the patients included peripheral edema,
pain, constipation, dyspnea and chest pain, impotenèe, and urinary
frequency. When the adverse events from this study were compared
to those observed during the first 24 weeks of daily injections of
leuprolide [6], no significant differences were observed. The two
formulations did not differ with respect to safety.
     All 10 patients in the pharmacokinetic study experienced
adverse events during the study. Events which occurred in more
than one patient included hot flashes, pain, constipation, and
rhinitis. All other events were reported in one patient each.

CONCLUSIONS

Leuprolide acetate as a depot injection appeared to be well
absorbed and provided steady and prolonged plasma drug
concentrations. The pharmacokinetic profile observed indicates
that the 7.5 mg depot formulation of leuprolide acetate is
suitable for administration as a monthly injection.
     The depot formulation of leuprolide acetate is as effective
in suppressing testosterone levels to well within the castrate
range, and in maintaining those levels, as daily 1mg subcutaneous
injection. Furthermore, there was no significant difference
between the objective response rates observed for the two dosage
forms, and the safety of the two formulations did not differ.

REFERENCES

1.   Johnson, E, Seeley, J, White, W and De Sombre, E (1976).
Endocrine-dependent rat mammary tumor regression: use of
gonadotropin releasing hormone analog. Science, 194, 329
2.   Robinson, MRG, Denis, L, Mahler, C, Walker, K, Stitch, R and
Lunglmayr, G (1985). An LH-RH analogue (Zoladex)in the management
of carcinoma of the prostate: a preliminary report comparing daily
subcutaneous injections with monthly depot injections. Eur J Surg
Oncol, 11, 159
3.   Walker, KJ, Turkes, AO, Turkes, A, Zwink, R, Beacock, C,
Buck, AC, Peeling, WB and Griffiths, K (1984). Treatment of
patients with advanced cancer of the prostate using a slow-release
(depot) formulation of the LHRH agonist ICI 118630 (Zoladex). J
Endocrinol, 103, R1
4.   Williams, G, Kerle, D, Griffin, S, Dunlop, H and Bloom, SR
(1984). Biodegradable polymer luteinising hormone releasing
hormone analogue for prostatic cancer: use of a new peptide
delivery system. Brit Med J, 289, 1580
5.   Schmidt, JD, Scott, WW, Gibbons, et al (1980). Chemotherapy
programs of the National Prostatic Cancer Project. Cancer, 45,
1937
6.   Garnick, MB, Glode, LM and The Leuprolide Study Group
(1984). Leuprolide versus diethylstilbestrol for metastatic
prostate cancer. New Engl J Med, 311, 1281

14

TREATMENT OF ADVANCED PROSTATIC CARCINOMAS BY AN LHRH ANALOGUE WITH OR WITHOUT AN ANTI-ANDROGEN

I. PAPADOPOULOS, F. SCHAUMKELL, H. BARTERMANN
and H. WAND

Urologische Universitätsklinik Kiel, Arnold-Heller-Strasse 7,
D-2300 Kiel 1, FRG

INTRODUCTION

Since the development of LHRH analogues an alternative has become available to the classical approach of castration for advanced carcinoma of the prostate. Numerous studies have verified the effect of such chemical castration on advanced carcinomas of the prostate [1-4]. LHRH analogues at supraphysiological doses reduce testicular testosterone biosynthesis [5]. The initial increased release of LH and FSH leads to an initial increase in testosterone levels. With continued administration, LHRH receptors in the hypophysis become blocked and the testosterone level falls within 4 weeks to castration values [6-10].

Clinical observations such as exacerbation of bone pain, increased impairment of urinary transport and a rise in prostatic acid phosphatase are indicative of the unfavourable influence of the initial rise in testosterone on the tumour [9,11,12]. In order to prevent this stimulation of the tumour during the initial phase and to achieve total elimination both of testicular and adrenal androgens, the latter being uninfluenced by the LHRH analogues, additional administration of anti-androgens (flutamide, anandrone) has been used [13]. They block intracellular testosterone or dihydrotestosterone receptors at the target organ, but lead to an increase in plasma testosterone. Other anti-androgens such as cyproterone acetate exert an additional inhibiting influence on testosterone synthesis via a centrally acting mechanism [14].

Habenicht et al. were able to show in animal experiments that an LHRH analogue combined with cyproterone exerts a clearly more intense inhibition of LH secretion and testosterone biosynthesis in the initial phase than the combination LHRH analogue plus flutamide [15].

Our clinical study was addressed to the as yet unanswered questions within the context of the ongoing controversy regarding the superiority of "complete androgen blockade" over conventional hormone therapy [16, 17]. The aims of this investigation were: 1. to compare the remission rates of LHRH monotherapy and combination with anti-androgens; 2. to evaluate the response of

LH, FSH, and testosterone concentrations during the initial phase
of the treatment; and finally to assess the frequency and severity
of side-effects.

PATIENTS AND METHODS

Over a period of 24 months 72 patients, ranging in age from 52 to
82 years (average age 71), with histologically confirmed prostatic
carcinomas (stage T3-4/N-/+/M-/+) were treated. Eighteen patients
(group A) were treated with an LHRH analogue (Decapeptyl[R],
Ferring GmbH, Kiel) as monotherapy, 31 (group B) with the
combination of LHRH and flutamide (Fugerel[R], Essex Pharma GmbH,
Munich) and 23 (Group C) with the combination of LHRH and
cyproterone acetate (Androcur[R], Schering, Berlin).
        Thirty-two patients (groups A#11, B#12, C#9) had advanced
carcinomas of the prostate with confirmed metastases (stage
T+N-/+/M-/+). Eight patients showed lymph node metastases
(T+N+Mo) demonstrated by computer tomography. Six patients showed
synchronous osseous and lymph node metastases (T+N+M1) (Table 1).

Table 1 Tumor stage of 72 patients with advanced prostatic
carcinomas (A = LHRH analogue, B = LHRH + flutamide, C = LHRH +
cyproterone acetate).

Stage	Group	n
13/4NoMo	A	7
	B	14
	C	11
T+N+Mo	A	–
	B	5
	C	3
T+NoM1	A	11
	B	12
	C	3
T+N+M1	A	–
	B	–
	C	6

Increased alkaline phosphatase was present in 20 patients (A:n=6,
B:n=7, C:n=7), increased prostatic acid phosphatase in 35 (A:n=8,
B:n=14, C:n=13).

Patients with carcinomas which had been previously treated or with secondary malignant carcinomas or were in poor general condition (WHO grade IV) were excluded from the study. The investigations on which the classification by disease stage was based are summarised in Table 2.

Table 2 Investigations for the clinical classification of tumors

---

Rectal palpation

Transrectal prostatic sonography

Prostate acid phosphatase (PAP-RIA) and alkaline phosphatase

Upper abdominal sonography

Thoracic X-ray on two planes

Inferior urogram

Skeletal scintigraphy/spot film radiography

Computer tomography

F = 3x 250 mg tablets Fugerel ®
A = 2x 50 mg tablets Androcur ®
♥ = 0,5 mg Decapeptyl ®   subcutaneously
♦ = 3,2 mg Decapeptyl ®   intramuscularly

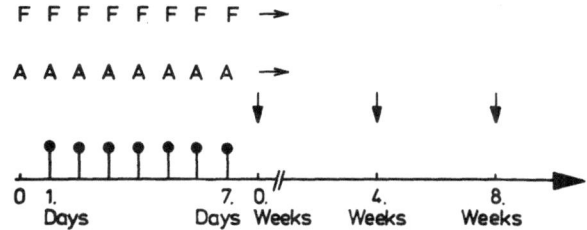

FIGURE 1 Therapeutic plan

In group A 0.5 mg of Decapeptyl^R as solution were injected subcutaneously every day for a 7-day period. On the 8th day 3.2 mg of the micro-encapsulated depot form were injected

151

intramuscularly. The depot form was given at 4-weekly intervals
(Fig. 1). In the combination therapy with Fugerel and with
Androcur administration of the anti-androgen commenced one day
before the first LHRH injection at dosage rates of 250 mg of
Fugerel and 50 mg of Androcur. Testosterone, FSH and LH were
determined before treatment was started, then daily from day 1
until day 15, then on days 21 and 30 and subsequently after 3 and
6 months. Alkaline and prostatic acid phosphatase were monitored
on days 5, 12 and 28 and after 3 and 6 months.
        In the 3rd and 6th months the volume of the prostate was
determined by transrectal prostatic sonography. To determine the
retrogression grading aspiration cytology was also carried out in
the 3rd and 6th months [18, 19].
        For assessment of the course of the disease or success of
the treatment the NPCP criteria were taken as a basis [12]. The
control investigations after 3 and 6 months, and optionally after
12, 18 and 24 months were carried out in accordance with Table 2.
If the patient responded to treatment the treatment was
continued. Alternatively, if, after 3 or 6 months, progression of
the tumours was established on the basis of the measurable
parameters, the treatment was changed. In the majority of cases,
where the general condition remained good, chemotherapy was
added. Where massive side-effects or severe cardiovascular
complications occurred the treatment was changed from that of
group B to group C, or vice versa, or discontinued. In some cases
objective signs of progression made change of therapy necessary
after as little as three months.

RESULTS

        The observation period of the 72 patients treated to date in
the three treatment groups has ranged from 12 to 24 months
(average 15 months). One patient in group A, who showed tumour
progression with massive formation of skeletal metastases died
within 6 months despite alternative chemotherapy with Estracyt.
One patient in group B and one in group C died of tumour cachexia
and a further 2 group C patients died from other causes (cardiac
decompensation). The cumulative progression curve of the patients
in the various treatment groups in relation to the occurrence of
the progression is shown in Fig. 2.
        Of the group A patients 6 showed partial remission, while in
2 patients the disease was stable. Progression was demonstrated
in 7 patients (Table 3). Of the group B patients, 20 of the 31
showed partial remission while in 4 the disease was stable
(Table 4). Group C showed partial remission in 8 and stability in
6, while progression was demonstrated in 9 out of the 23 patients
(Table 5). In 6 out of 8 group A patients with raise of prostatic
phosphatase normalisation of the phosphatases recurred during
therapy within 6 months. In Fugerel group B prostatic phosphatase
levels normalised in 12 out of 14, and in group C in 9 out of 13
patients. Plasma testosterone values in group A, after an initial

152

Table 3 Assessment of 18 patients (LHRH group) with prostatic carcinomas in accordance with the NPCP criteria. CR = complete remission, PR = partial remission, S = stable condition, P = progression.

Criteria	Stage T+NoMo n = 7	T+NoM1 n = 11
CR	–	–
PR	5	4
S	1	1
P	1	6

rise, were brought down below 0.5 ng/ml within 4 weeks (Fig. 3). Group C a more rapid fall in plasma testosterone within 2 weeks was observed (Fig. 4) whereas in group B testosterone did not fall to castration levels until after 12 weeks (Fig. 5). Serum concentrations of FSH and LH remained in the subnormal range throughout treatment in all groups. A rapid reduction in volume (over 30% after 3 months) by transrectal prostatic sonography with normalisation of the echo structure was observable in about 60% of patients from all groups.

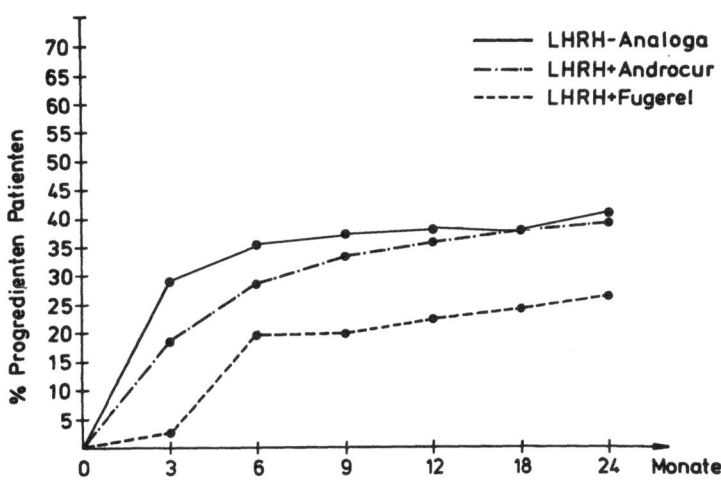

FIGURE 2 Cumulative progression curve of the patient in the three group

Table 4 Assessment of 31 patients (Decapeptyl + Fugerel) with prostate carcinomas according to the NPCP criteria. CR = complete remission, PR = partial remission, S = stable condition, P = progression.

Criteria	Stage	T+NoMo n = 14	T+N+Mo n = 6	T+NoM+ n = 11
CR		-	-	-
PR		12	3	5
S		1	1	2
P		1	2	4

Table 5 Assessment of 23 patients (Androcur) with prostate carcinomas according to the NPCP criteria. CR = complete remission, PR = partial remission, S = stable condition, P = progression.

Criteria	Stage	T+NoMo n = 11	T+N+Mo n = 2	T+NoM+ n = 3	T+N+M+ n = 6
CR		-	-	-	-
PR		6	1	-	1
S		3	1	1	1
P		2	1	2	4

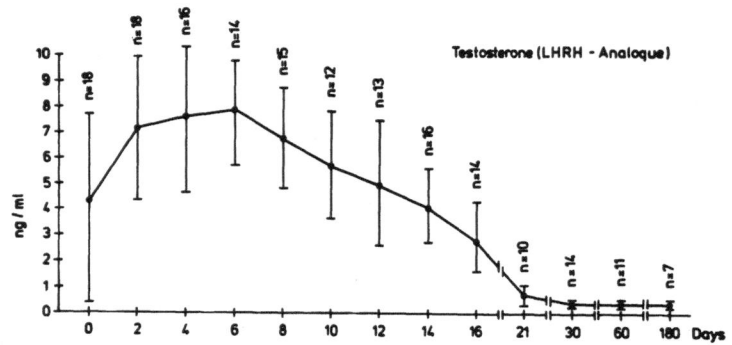

FIGURE 3   Plasma testosterone levels in Arm A (LHRH-analogue group)

SIDE-EFFECTS

In all sexually active men testosterone suppression produced loss
of libido and capacity for erection. Hot flushes of varying
extent were recorded in 65% of all patients within 3 weeks after
the starting of therapy. In 15% of patients in the Fugerel group

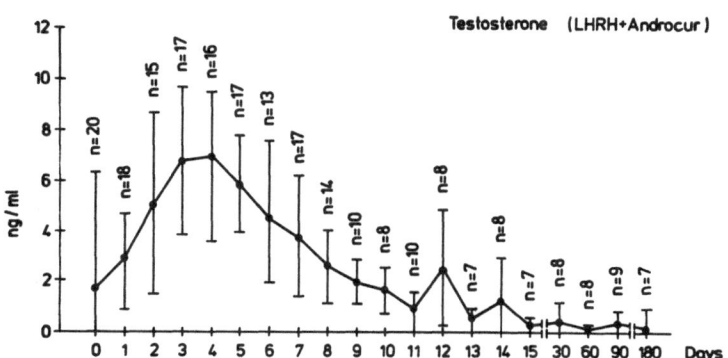

FIGURE 4 Testosterone levels in Arm C (Decapeptyl + Androcur)

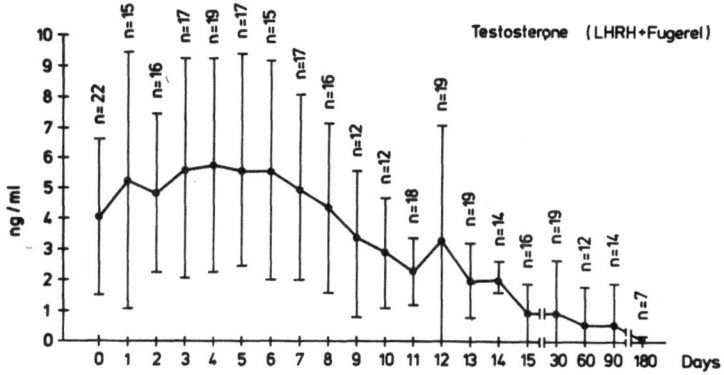

FIGURE 5 Plasma testosterone levels in Arm B (Decapeptyl +
Fugerel)

gastro-intestinal disorders occurred. In the Androcur group,
despite remission, 2 cases of death through cardiac insufficiency
were observed.

DISCUSSION

Following practically complete elimination of testicular androgens by administration of an LHRH analogue the remission rate with prostatic carcinomas in our own patients was 61%. Remission rates in the literature are between 60 and 80% [1,3,6,11,20]. With a combination of an LHRH analogue and an anti-androgen it was possible moreover, to block production of adrenal androgens thereby achieving the maximum hormonal effect. The initial testosterone rise produced by LHRH agonists with exacerbation of the tumour and worsening of the clinical symptoms should be suppressed by administration of anti-androgens. In clinical studies differences were observed in respect of the 18 months survival rate between a combination of an LHRH analogue and a pure anti-androgen (flutamide or anandrone) (97%) or orchiectomy plus cyproterone acetate (70%) [21, 22].

In 61% of patients treated with Decapeptyl[R] as monotherapy in the present study clinical remission was observed. In all patients plasma testosterone values, after a brief rise, fell within 4 weeks to castration level and thereafter, during the period of observation, showed no further rise. In no patient in the LHRH monotherapy group was there an exacerbation of bone pain or a rise in prostatic acid phosphatase. In the Fugerel group clinical remission was observed in 77.5% of patients. Plasma testosterone values fell to castration levels within 12 weeks and thereafter did not rise again. Up to the point where the castration level was reached no deterioration in the clinical symptoms was observed in any of the patients. In the majority of the patients in spite of only slowly falling serum testosterone levels there occurred an improvement in the clinical symptoms.

In 60.8% of patients who received Androcur plus LHRH treatment clinical remission was observed. Plasma testosterone values in this group, after an initial rise within 2 weeks, then fell to castration levels.

In all treated patients loss of libido and potency occurred, while 60% suffered hot flushes which continued over a period of months. In 15% of the patients treated with Fugerel gastro-intestinal side-effects were observed and as a result of these therapy had to be discontinued or changed in 4 patients. In the Androcur group 2 deaths were observed as a result of cardiac insufficiency despite a good therapeutic effect.

By means of this study and despite the small number of patients involved it was possible to show that the addition of flutamide administration in comparison with the LHRH analogue as monotherapy or in combination with cyproterone acetate yielded better results. The height of the testosterone level in the initial phase seems to be without negative influence either on the clinical symptoms or on the subsequent development of the tumour. The incorporation of cyproterone acetate in the LHRH analogue therapy however, in view of the high incidence of side-effects, high cost and doubtful therapeutic effect, is not to be recommended.

REFERENCES

1.   Papadopoulos, I, Kleinschmidt, K and Weissbach, L (1986). Akt Urol, 17, 315

2.   Pressant, CA, Solonay, MS and Klioze, SS (1985). Cancer, 56, 2416

3.   Seppelt, U, Bertermann, H and Saerbeck, Ch (1986). Urologe, A, 25, 298

4.   Wenderoth, UK and Jacobi, GH (1985). World J Urol, 1, 40

6.   Borgmann, V, Nagel, R, Schmidt-Gollwitzer, M. and Hardt, W (1982). Akt Urol, 13, 200

7.   Pinto, H, Wajckenberg, BL, Lima, FB, Goldman, J, Comeru-Schally, AM and Schally, AV (1979). Acta Endocrinol, 91, 1

8.   Sandow, J, von Rechenberg, W, Jerzabek, G, Engelbart, K, Kuhl, H and Fraser H (1980). Acta Endocrinol, 94, 489

9.   Santen, RJ and Warner, B (1985). Urology, 25, 53

10.   Schally, AV, Redding, TW, and Comaru-Schally, AM (1983). The Prostate, 4, 545

11.   Faure, N. Lemay, A, Laroche B, Robert, G, Plante, R, Jean, C, Thabet, M, Roy, R and Fazekas, AT (1983). The Prostate, 4, 601

12.   Tolis G, and Koutsillieris, M (1985). Das Forgeschritene Prostatakarzinon: Eine therapeutische Herausforderung. In: Labrie, F and Wenderoth, UK (Eds.). "Eine neue Strategie bei der Behandlung des Prostatakarzinoms" Buserelin (Suprefact)". p.36. (Exerpta Medica: Amsterdam).

13.   Pont, A, William PL and Loose, DA (1982). Ann Intern Med, 97, 370

14.   Walsh, PC and Korenmann, SG (1971). J. Urol, 105, 850

15.   Habenicht, FU, Witthaus, E and Neumann, F (1986). Akt Urol, 17, 10

18.   Leistenschneidor, W and Nagel, R (1983). Urologa A, 22, 144

19.   Leistenschneider, W and Nagel, R (1980). Akt Urol, 11, 263

20.   Wenderoth, UK and Jacobi, GH (1985). Akt Urol, 16, 58

21.   Gluliani, L, Pescatore, D and Gilberti, C (1980). Eur J Urol, 6, 145

22.   Labrie, F, Dupont, A, and Belanger, A (1985). Complete androgen blockade for the treatment of prostatic cancer. In: DeVita, VT, Hellmann, S and Rosenberg, SA (Eds.). "Important Advances in Oncology". p. 193. (Lippincott, Philadelphia)

15

THE USE OF GnRH ANALOGUES IN OVARIAN CANCER

G. EMONS, G.S. PAHWA, R. STRUM, R. KNUPPEN and F. OBERHEUSER

Klinik für Frauenheilkunde und Geburtshilfe, Institut für Biochemische Endokrinologie Medizinische Universität zu Lübeck, D-2400 Lübeck, FRG

INTRODUCTION

In Western Europe and the USA ovarian carcinomata are one of the most common causes of cancer deaths in women. Though there have been some advances in surgical, radio-, and cytotoxic-chemotherapy, the overall results of the treatment of this disease are still unsatisfactory. In addition, modern aggressive chemotherapy is accompanied by severe side effects. Therefore, an actual trend in oncology has been to reduce at least therapy- induced morbidity, if its efficacy cannot be significantly increased by more aggressive regimes. In the treatment of breast- and endometrial cancer this has been partially achieved by the introduction of additive or ablative hormonal treatments, taking advantage of the sex-steroid dependence of a large number of these tumors, which is reflected by the presence of receptors for oestrogens and/or progestins. Also in ovarian carcinomata sex-steroid receptors have been found [1]. Attempts at endocrine treatment of ovarian cancer, however, using either progestins or antioestrogens have hitherto not accumulated convincing evidence for the effectiveness of this approach [1].
    Epidemiological observations suggest that the risk of ovarian carcinoma decreases with the number of pregnancies and the duration of the use of oral contraceptives [2,3]. One explanation for this phenomenon is that frequent ovulations rupturing the coelomic epithelium may lead to the development of ovarian cancer [4]. Another explanation is that the formation and proliferation of ovarian carcinomata might be dependent on a direct action of luteinizing hormone (LH) and follicle stimulating hormone (FSH) on the tumor cells. Thus the decrease of LH- and FSH-secretion associated with pregnancies and the use of oral contraceptives might be the mechanism conferring some protection against ovarian cancer. This "gonadotropin theory" is further supported by the fact that the incidence of ovarian carcinomata rises steeply with the advent of the menopause, when gonadotropin secretion is physiologically increased. If the development and progression of ovarian cancer were LH- and FSH-dependent, a suppression of

these gonadotropins, nowadays most effectively achieved by GnRH
analogues, might be beneficial for patients suffering from the
disease.

Recently, direct effects of GnRH agonists on human breast
cancer have been postulated [5,6]. In vitro experiments
demonstrated that the proliferation of certain breast cancer
cell lines can be inhibited by GnRH agonists [7] or GnRH
antagonists [8]. Though these results are at present
controversial [9], gonadotropin-releasing hormone binding sites
could be characterized in breast cancer tissue and cell lines
[8]. Also evidence for the production of GnRH in these cells
has been accumulated suggesting an autocrine regulation of the
tumors by this GnRH-system [10]. If a similar system,
involving either GnRH or GnRH-like activity was present in
human ovarian malignancies, another point might exist for the
therapeutic use of GnRH analogues in this disease.

Thus, the application of GnRH analogues in patients with
ovarian cancer could be beneficial via two mechanisms: 1)
suppression of LH- and FSH-secretion, thus removing a possible
proliferation stimulus, 2) direct inhibitory effects on the
tumor cells mediated by putative receptors for GnRH or
GnRH-like peptides.

EFFECTS OF GnRH AGONIST-INDUCED SUPPRESSION OF GONADOTROPINS ON THE PROLIFERATION OF OVARIAN CANCER

Apart from the above mentioned epidemiological data, suggesting
a gonadotropin dependence of ovarian malignancies, several
animal and receptor studies have provided data in favour of
this theory. In experimental tumors, obtained by intrasplenic
autotransplanta- tion of ovaries in castrated rats, Kullander
[11] could prevent growth by the application of the GnRH
agonist [D-Trp^6]GnRH (Decapeptyl). With the same GnRH
analogue, the growth of the human ovarian carcinoma line
OVCAR-3 in nude mice could be inhibited [12].
LH(hCG)-receptors could be demonstrated in some malignant
tumors of the human ovary [13]. The proliferation of ovarian
cancer cell lines in vivo could be stimulated by human
gonadotropins [14,15]. Initial clinical trials have shown that
the reduction of LH and FSH by [D-Trp^6]GnRH can induce
partial remission or lead to stable disease in patients with
advanced ovarian cancer relapsing after conventional treatment
[11,16,17].

These experimental and clinical observations motivated us
to initiate a prospective, randomized, placebo-controlled study
on the usefulness of GnRH agonist-induced suppression of LH and
FSH in patients with ovarian cancer. This multicentre clinical
study, prepared by Prof. Kullander from Malmö, Sweden and us,
was planned in detail and carried out by the colleagues listed
in Appendix 1.

The study is being carried out with patients in whom an
advanced ovarian cancer (FIGO Stage III or IV) has been
diagnosed for the first time. After surgical treatment and

staging, the patients volunteering for the study (informed
consent), were randomized into a Decapeptyl group and the
placebo group. All patients will received a standardized first
line polychemotherapy (containing cis-platinum). Decapeptyl or
placebo administration were additional and will be continued if
a second line chemotherapy becomes necessary (Fig. 1). The
study will be carried out in a double blind manner.

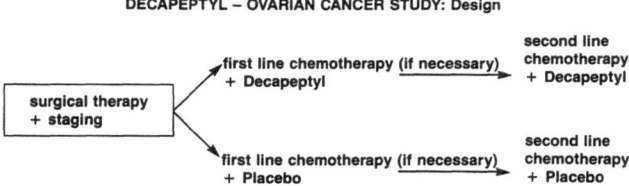

DECAPEPTYL – OVARIAN CANCER STUDY: Design

FIGURE 1   Design of ovarian cancer study

        The criteria for entry in the study are given in
Table 2. Additional endocrine therapy (e.g. antioestrogens,
progestins) is not allowed.

Table 2   Decapeptyl-ovarian cancer study - entry criteria

- Ovarian cancer stage FIGO III/IV, diagnosed by surgical and
  histological staging.

- Patients are eligible for first line chemotherapy,
  containing cis-platinum.

- Informed consent (including randomization)

- No other malignancy

- No other endocrine therapy

        Decapeptyl or placebo administration (Table 3) starts
within 2 weeks after surgical therapy and will be continued for
at least 2 years or until the death of the patient. A
follow-up period of at least 2 more years is planned. At least
100 patients shall be recruited for each, the Decapeptyl and
the placebo group.

Table 3 Decapeptyl-ovarian cancer study - Decapeptyl regimen

Starting within 14 days after the operation:

7 days: 500 µg Decapeptyl s.c./day
day 8:   3 mg Decapeptyl depot i.m. repeated every 28 days

Control group:

7 days: saline s.c.
day 8:   peptide-free microcarrier suspension i.m. repeated
         every 28 days

The main parameter of the study will be survival time.
An effect of the Decapeptyl therapy will be accepted, if in the
treatment group, survival times are at least 20% longer than in
the control group.

Other parameters that are monitored but not analyzed
statistically are given in Table 4.

Table 4 Decapeptyl-ovarian cancer study - parameters to be
assessed

Main Study Parameters: Survival time after primary operation

Other Study Parameters: - remission rates
                          - relapse free interval
                          - duration of response
                          - duration of survival
                          - toxicity

A stratification according to histological types of the
malignancies will be carried out (Table 5). At regular
intervals (approx. 6 months) preliminary evaluations of the
study results will be performed. If the Decapeptyl group have
significantly longer survival times before the end of the
recruitment or follow-up phase, the control group will be also
treated with Decapeptyl. The study will be stopped if the
Decapeptyl group performs significantly worse than the control
group or when severe side-effects with high frequency have been
observed.

Table 5 Decapeptyl-ovarian cancer study - stratification

Serous cystadenocarcinoma   stratum I

Mucinous cystadenocarcinoma
Endometrioid carcinoma   stratum II
Clear cell carcinoma
Undifferentiated carcinoma
Malignant Brenner Tumor

Granulosa cell tumor
Thecal cell tumor   stratum III
Gynandroblastoma
Androblastoma

    This study was started for the German participants in
October 1987. The Scandinavian groups will enter the study
during 1988.
    No results can be presented at the moment, but we are
confident that at the end of the study we shall be able to
provide a definite statement whether or not GnRH-agonist
treatment is effective in the therapy of ovarian cancer.

DIRECT EFFECTS OF GnRH ANALOGUES ON HUMAN OVARIAN CARCINOMATA

In rats, GnRH has been described as a modulator of ovarian
functions [18,19]. In this species, high affinity, low
capacity receptors have been demonstrated in the ovaries,
comparable to the pituitary GnRH receptors [18,19]. Also in
the human, direct inhibitory effects of a GnRH agonist on a
hormone-producing ovarian tumour (arrhenoblastoma) [20] and on
granulosa cell progesterone secretion [21] have been shown.
High affinity, low capacity GnRH receptors, however, could not
be found in human ovarian tissue [22]. In later studies, low
affinity, high capacity GnRH binding sites have been
characterized in human corpora lutea [23,24].
    As a first step to elucidate possible direct effects of
GnRH analogues on human ovarian cancer, we checked whether or
not GnRH-binding sites are present in these tumors. Using
^{125}I-[D- Ala^6,des Gly^{10}]GnRH ethylamide as labelled
ligand, we were able to demonstrate low affinity, high capacity
binding of this GnRH-agonist (GnRH-A) in membranes from a
number of human ovarian epithelial carcinomata [25]. This
binding was temperature and time dependent, the best conditions
being incubation at $0°C$ for 6 hours. The GnRH-A binding was a
linear function of plasma membrane concentration over a range
of 200-1200 µg protein/ tube. Protein concentrations between
390 and 1560 µg/tube produced nearly parallel inhibition
curves [25].

The analysis of binding data obtained from inhibition curves with unlabelled [D-Ala[6],des Gly[10]]GnRH ethylamide, using a ligand program [26] was consistent with a single class of low affinity, high capacity binding sites (K_a = 1.42 ± 0.14 x 10 M $^{5-1}$ (x ± SE), R = 69 ± 69 x 10^{-12} M/Mg membrane protein, n=32).

The specificity of the GnRH binding site was tested using other peptides in concentrations up to 10^{-4}M. Oxytocin, thyrotropin-releasing hormone, and corticotropin-releasing factor did not cause any displacement of ^{125}I-GnRH-A. Somatostatin, however, showed crossreactivity in some of the tumors tested, whereas it did not displace the GnRH-A in others. Native GnRH and the GnRH-antagonist [D-p-Glu[1],D-Phe[2],D-Trp[3,6]]GnRH were bound with nearly the same characteristics as the GnRH agonist (K_a=0.65 ± 0.15 x 10^5M^{-1} native GnRH, n=4; and 0.62 ± 0.21 x 10^5M^{-1} for the antagonist, n=3).

Of the 40 ovarian epithelial carcinomata tested, GnRH-A binding could be demonstrated in 32. Table 6 gives the binding characteristics of 10 representative ovarian malignancies analyzed.

Using the same binding assay [25], we were able to measure binding sites of the same characteristics in human term placentae, human corpora lutea and human granulosa cells. With a similar system Iwashita et al [27] characterized a comparable binding site in human chorionic villi and term placenta (K_a for [D-Ala[6], des Gly[10]]GnRH ethylamide=5.4 x 10^5M^{-1}). Currie et al [28]

Table 6   GnRH binding sites in a selection of human ovarian carcinomata [25]

Material	Binding Sites [10^{-12}M/mg MP^a]	K_a [10^5M^{-1}]
Highly differentiated serous cystadenocarcinoma	76	1.4
Poorly differentiated solid adenocarcinoma	16	2.3
Poorly differentiated serous adenocarcinoma	212	0.8
Highly differentiated serous papillary adenocarcinoma	148	1.5
Poorly differentiated serous papillary adenocarcinoma	177	1.4

Poorly differentiated adenopapillary carcinoma	97	1.5
Highly differentiated serous papillary adenocarcinoma	301	1.7
Partly differentiated endometroid adenocarcinoma	330	1.0
Poorly differentiated adenocarcinoma	n.d.[b]	n.d.
Partly differentiated partly mucinous adenocarcinoma	n.d.	n.d.

[a]MP = membrane protein, [b]not detected.

found a higher K_a for both native GnRH (K_a=6.2 x 10^7M^{-1}) and [D-Ser(TBU)[6]]LHRH ethylamide (K_a=5.5 x 10^7M^{-1}). Bramley et al [24] from the same laboratory described a similar GnRH-A-binding site in human corpora lutea (K_a=3 x 10^7M^{-1}). The reason for the lower affinities observed in our system and by Iwashita et al [27] as compared to those by Currie et al [28] and Bramley et al [24] are probably due to differences in the binding assays used. Thus, we assume that the GnRH-binding site in human epithelial ovarian carcinomata is the same as the one in human granulosa cells, human corpora lutea and human placental tissue. A similar low affinity/high capacity binding site for GnRH with a K_a in the order of 10^6M^{-1} has been described by Eidne et al [10] in human breast cells. These authors stress the point that the breast cancer site has similar affinities for native GnRH, GnRH agonists, and GnRH antagonists, while pituitary GnRH receptors have a significantly higher affinity for the analogues than for native GnRH. The same observation was made for the GnRH binding site in human placental tissue [29] and the GnRH-binding site characterized by us in ovarian carcinomata.

At present, the functional importance of the GnRH binding site in human ovarian cancer is still obscure. In breast cancer and placental tissue these low affinity GnRH-binding sites have been interpreted as receptors for locally produced GnRH or GnRH- related peptides and direct effects of GnRH analogues in these tissues have been demonstrated [10,27]. However, the properties of the placental and breast cancer GnRH binding sites are clearly distinct from those of the pituitary GnRH receptor, possibly reflecting the need for a low affinity interaction when the regulatory ligand is produced in abundance at close proximity to its receptor sites. Thus, direct effects of GnRH agonists or antagonists on human breast cancer [8] and placental [23] cells have been achieved with rather high (10^{-6}-10^{-5}M) concentrations of GnRH analogues. Another hypothesis might be that the natural ligand, produced locally, might have a much higher affinity for its receptor than pituitary GnRH and its analogues.

The question whether GnRH or a GnRH-like peptide is produced in human ovarian cancer cells as a part of an autocrine regulatory mechanism remains to be elucidated. A first step is the demonstration of the functional role of the binding sites. This could be done by studying the effects of GnRH agonists and antagonists on the proliferation of ovarian cancer cells in vitro and whether or not second messenger mechanisms are activated in the cells by GnRH and its analogues. These studies are presently being performed in our laboratory.

It cannot be ruled out that the GnRH binding sites in ovarian carcinomata may represent only a phylogenetic residue without functional importance. But even in this case it should be interesting to look for a correlation between GnRH binding site density, the histology of the tumors and the clinical course of the disease. In addition, a correlation with hCG receptors (in cooperation with Prof. Rajaiemi, Oulu, Finland) will be performed. Also a further biochemical characterization of the binding site is necessary and presently is being performed in our laboratory.

CONCLUSIONS

Research on the use of GnRH analogues in human ovarian cancer has just started. Thus, only few hard clinical and experimental data can be reported at present. The evidence, however, available today supplies convincing motivation for intensive research, both experimental and clinical on the putative use of GnRH analogues in the treatment of this fatal disease. The result of this work might be that GnRH analogue therapy is free of severe side effects but also free of significant effects on tumor growth. The chance, however, of developing a non-toxic therapy with beneficial effects in patients with ovarian cancer, obliges us to accept this challenge.

ACKNOWLEDGEMENTS

The multi-center clinical study on the effects of Decapeptyl in advanced ovarian cancer is supported by Ferring Arzneimittel GmbH, Kiel, F.R.G. The experimental research on GnRH binding sites in human epithelial ovarian carcinoma has been supported by the Deutsche Forschungsgemeinschaft (SFB 232/C2) and will be sponsored by Ferring, Kiel. Dr. G.S. Pahwa receives a research grant from the Alexander v. Humbodlt-Foundation and is on deputation from Regional Research Laboratory (C.S.I.R.) Jammu-Tawi 180001, India. We are grateful to the Biomedical Computing Technology Information Center, Vanderbilt Medical Center, Nashville, Tennessee, for the supply of the Ligand-program.

REFERENCES

1. Desombre, ER, Holt, JA and Herbst, AL (1987). Steroid receptors in breast, uterine, and ovarian malignancy. In Gold, JJ and Josimovich, JB (eds.) "Gynecologic Endocrinology". p.511. (New York: Plenum Publishing Corporation)
2. Casagrande, JT, Louie, EW, Pike, MC, Roy, S, Rock, RK and Henderson, BE (1979). Incessant ovulation and ovarian cancer. Lancet, 2, 170
3. Wynder, LE, Dodo, H and Barber, RK (1969). Epidemiology of cancer of the ovary. Cancer, 23, 352
4. Fathalla, MF (1971). Incessant ovulation - a factor in ovarian neoplasia? Lancet, 2, 163
5. Manni, A, Santen, R, Harvey, H, Lipton, A and Max, D (1986). Treatment of breast cancer with gonadotropin-releasing hormone. Endocr Rev, 7, 89
6. Nicholson, RI, Walker, KJ, Turkes, A, Dyas, J, Plowman, PN, Williams, M and Blamley, RW (1985). Endocrinological and clinical aspects of LHRH action (ICI 118630) in hormone dependent breast cancer. J Steroid Biochem, 23, 843
7. Miller, WR, Scott, WN, Morris, R, Fraser, HM and Sharpe, RM (1985). Growth of human breast cancer cells inhibited by a luteinizing hormone-releasing hormone agonist. Nature, 313, 231
8. Eidne, KA, Flanagan, CA, Harris, NS and Millar, RP (1987). Gonadotropin-releasing hormone (GnRH)-binding sites in human breast cancer cell lines and inhibitory effects of GnRH antagonists. J Clin Endocrinol Metab, 64, 425
9. Wilding, G, Chen, M and Gelman, EP (1987). LHRH agonist and human breast cancer cells. Nature. 329, 770
10. Eidne, KA, Harris, NS, Millar, RP and Wilcox, J (1987). GnRH-immunoreactivity and GnRH-mRNA in two human breast cancer cell lines MDA-MB-231 and ZR-75-1. Program of 69th Annual Meeting of the Endocrine Society, June 10-12, Indianapolis, Abstract 653
11. Kullander, S (1986). LH-RH agonist treatment in ovarian cancer. Eur J Cancer Clin Oncol, 22, 724
12. Mortel, R, Satyaswaroop, PG, Schally, AV, Hamilton, T and Ozols, R (1986). Inhibitory effect of GnRH superagonist on the growth of human ovarian carcinoma NIH: OVCAR 3 in the nude mouse. Program of Annual Meeting Society of Gynecologic Oncology, Abstract
13. Rajanniemi, H, Kauppila, A, Rönnberg, L, Selander, K and Pystynen, P (1981). LH(hCG) receptors in benign and malignant tumors of human ovary. Acta Obstet Gynecol Scand (Suppl), 101, 83
14. Simon, WE and Hölzel, F (1979). Hormone sensitivity of gynecological tumor cells in tissue cultures. J Cancer Res Clin Oncol, 94, 307
15. Simon, WE, Albrecht, M, Hänsel, M, Dietl, M and Hölzel, F (1983). Cell lines derived from human ovarian carcinomas: growth stimulation by gonadotropic and steroid hormones. J Natl Cancer Inst, 70, 839

16.   Parmar, H, Nicoll, J, Stockdale, A, Cassoni, A, Phillips, RH, Lightman, SL and Schally, AV (1985). Advanced ovarian carcinoma: response to the agonist D-Trp^6-LH-RH. Cancer Treat Rep, 69, 1341

17.   Parmar, H, Phillips, RH, Rustin, G, Lucas, C, Schally AV and Lightman, SL (1987). Response to D-Trp^6-LHRH (Decapeptyl) in ovarian cancer. J Steroid Biochem (Suppl), 28, 66A

18.   Knecht, M, Ranta, T, Feng, P, Shinohara, O and Catt, KJ (1985). Gonadotropin-releasing hormone as a modulator of ovarian function. J Steroid Biochem, 23, 771

19.   Hsueh, AJW and Schaeffer, M (1985). Gonadotropin-releasing hormone as a paracrine hormone and neurotransmitter in extrapituitary sites. J Steroid Biochem, 23, 757

20.   Lamberts, SWJ, Timmers, JM, Osterom, R, Verleun, T, Rommerts, FG and DeJong, FH (1982). Testosterone secretion by cultured arrhenoblastoma cells: suppression by a luteinizing hormone-releasing hormone agonist. J Clin Endocrinol Metab, 54, 450

21.   Tureck, RW, Mastroianni, L Jr, Blasco, L and Strauss, JF III (1982). Inhibition of human granulosa cell progesterone secretion by a gonadotropin-releasing hormone agonist. J Clin Endocrinol Metab, 54, 1078

22.   Clayton, RN and Huhtaniemi, I (1982). Absence of gonadotropin-releasing hormone receptors in human gonadal tissue. Nature, 299, 56

23.   Popkin, R, Bramley, TA, Currie, A, Shaw, RW, Baird, DT and Fraser, HM (1983). Specific binding of luteinizing hormone releasing hormone to human luteal tissue. Biochem Biophys Res Commun, 114, 750

24.   Bramley, TA, Menzies, GS and Baird, DT (1985). Specific binding of gonadotrophin-releasing hormone and an agonist to human corpus luteum homogenates: characterization, properties, and luteal phase levels. J Clin Endocrinol Metab, 61, 834

25.   Emons, G, Pahwa, GS, Brack, C, Sturm, R, Oberheuser, F and Knuppen, R (1988). Gonadotropin-releasing hormone binding sites in human epithelial ovarian carcinomata. J Clin Endocrinol Metab, submitted

26.   Clayton, RN, Shakespear, RA. Duncan, JA and Marshall, JD (with appendix by Munson, PJ and Rodbard, D) (1979). Radioiodinated nondegradable gonadotropin-releasing hormone analogs: new probes for the investigation of pituitary gonadotropin-releasing hormone receptors. Endocrinology, 105, 1369

27.   Iwashita, M, Evans, MI and Catt, KJ (1986). Characteriza- tion of a gonadotropin-releasing hormone receptor site in term placenta and chorionic villi. J Clin Endocrinol Metab, 62, 127

28.   Currie, AJ, Fraser, HM and Sharpe, RM (1981). Human placental receptors for luteinizing hormone releasing hormone. Biochem Biophys Res Commun, 89, 332

29.   Belisle, S, Guevin, JF, Bellabarba, D and Lehoux, JG
(1984).   Luteinizing hormone-releasing hormone binds to
enriched human placental membranes and stimulates in vitro the
synthesis of bioactive human chorionic gonadotropin.   J Clin
Endocrinol Metab, <u>59</u>, 119

Appendix   Decapeptyl-ovarian cancer study - participants

Prof. Nieminen	University of Helsinki, Finland
Prof. Kauppila	University of Oulu, Finland
Prof. Kullander	University of Lund, Malmö, Sweden
Dr. Jeppson	University of Lund, Malmö, Sweden
Prof. Skryten	Dept. of Ob/Gyn, Stavanger, Norway
Prof. Krebs	University of Bonn, F.R.G.
Dr. Werner	University of Bonn, F.R.G.
Prof. Jütting	Kreiskrankenhaus Eutin, F.R.G.
Dr. Austermann	Kreiskrankenhaus Eutin, F.R.G.
Prof. Semm	University of Kiel, F.R.G.
Prof. Mettler	University of Kiel, F.R.G.
Dr. Mayer-Eichberger	University of Kiel, F.R.G.
Prof. Oberheuser	Med. University of Lübeck, F.R.G.
Dr. Emons	Med. University of Lübeck, F.R.G.
Prof. Ohlenroth	Women's Hospital Osnabrück, F.R.G.
Dr. Gethmann	Women's Hospital Osnabrück, F.R.G.
Prof. Löhrs (Ref. Pathologist)	Inst. of Pathology, Med. Univers. of Lübeck, F.R.G.
Prof. Fassl, Dr. Mehring (Documentation and Statistical Evaluation)	Inst. for Medical statistics and Documentation, Med. Univers. of Lübeck, F.R.G.

16
GnRH ANALOGUES IN THE TREATMENT OF OVARIAN CARCINOMA

W. JÄGER, L. WILDT and N. LANG
Department of Gynecology and Obstetrics,
University of Erlangen-Nürnberg, D-8520 Erlangen, FRG

INTRODUCTION

Bast and coworkers described in 1981 a high-molecular weight glycoprotein, which was defined by reactivity with the murine monoclonal antibody OC-125 and which they named CA-125 [1]. CA-125 is expressed in high amounts by neoplastic ovarian tissue and can also be detected in the serum of patients with ovarian carcinoma [2-4]. Its importance for surveilance of these patients is based on the observation that an increase of CA-125 serum levels is always associated with a progression of disease [5, 6]. However, the patho-physiological function of the glycoprotein and the factors determining its serum levels are still unknown. Because a massive increase of CA-125 serum levels has been described in patients developing ovarian hyperstimulation syndrome as a consequence of treatment with exogenous gonadotropins we supposed that CA-125 serum levels are in some way controlled by the gonadotropins [7]. The demonstration of an increase of CA-125 serum levels during the menstrual cycle in healthy women parallel to the follicular development was in keeping with that hypothesis. This increase of CA-125 serum levels could be abolished by the blockade of follicular maturation by hormonal contraceptives [8].
It was therefore tempting to speculate that even the increase of CA-125 serum levels observed in patients with progressive ovarian cancer could be explained by a similar mechanism. To test this hypothesis we have used the GnRH agonist Decapeptyl to suppress pituitary gonadotropin secretion in such patients.

MATERIAL AND METHODS

Patients

A total of 33 patients have been studied since August 1985. All patients had previously been operated on for advanced ovarian cancer and were pretreated with differing chemotherapy regimens containing cisplatinum and alkylating agents [9].

Twentytwo of these patients who had been referred to our hospital since February 1986 participated in the present study and received the agonist treatment. Eleven patients who developed relapses between August 1985, when we initiated serial CA-125 determinations, and February 1986 remained untreated and were considered as controls. Increasing CA-125 serum levels were observed in all patients during progression of disease or recurrent tumor growth. All patients were in a condition at that time, where all established treatment modalities were exhausted. For this same reason all but one patient were not subjected to any major diagnostic procedure except rectal or vaginal palpation and ultrasonography. In that one patient we performed a third tumor reduction in January 1988.

GnRH Agonist administration

The GnRH agonist [D-Trp^6]LHRH (Decapeptyl, Ferring GmbH, Kiel, FRG) was available in two application forms for intramuscular injection. For daily injections a solution containing 0.1mg of the peptide and for monthly injections 3.2mg of the microencapsulated form were used [10]. The microencapsulated slow-release form was prepared by mixing the dry powdery substance with 2ml of dispersion solution by rapid push and pull maneouvres using two connected syringes.
  In the first 5 patients daily injections of the 0.1mg preparation were given for 28 days, thereafter the slow-release form was administered every 26-28 days. All other patients received the 3.2mg dose from the beginning. In three patients the interval between injections was shortened to 14 days based on the results of the FSH and LH determinations.
  Most of treatment was performed on an outpatient basis at the Department of Obstetrics and Gynecology of the University of Erlangen. In 6 patients the injections and blood samplings were continued after 4 months by a gynecologist near their home.

GnRH-challenge test

A GnRH test was performed in 7 patients after half a year of treatment. It was repeated when a sudden increase of CA-125 concentrations was detected or FSH or LH serum levels failed to decline or increased. Blood samples were obtained every 15 minutes starting 30 minutes before iv injection of 100µg LH-RH (LH-RH Ferring, Ferring Gmbh, Kiel, FRG) and finished 120 minutes thereafter.

CA-125, FSH and LH determinations

Blood samples were drawn from all patients before injection of Decapeptyl. Follicle stimulating hormone (FSH) and luteinizing hormone (LH) were measured with immunoradiometric assays using monoclonal antibodies (FSH MAIA CLONE, LH MAIA CLONE, Serono, Freiburg, FRG). The range of the standard curve extended from 0.5mIU/ml to 150mIU/ml for FSH and 0.5mIU/ml to 200mIU/ml for

LH (2nd IRP 78-549 - FSH; 1st IRP 68-40 - LH). Inter-and intraassay coefficients of variation were below 6%. Sera were assayed in duplicate for their CA-125 content by an immunoradiometric assay using the monoclonal OC-125 as catcher and tracer (ELSA-CA-125, ID-CIS, Dreieich, FRG). The range of the standard curve extended from 6 to 500 U/ml. Samples with concentrations above the upper limit of the assay were reassayed after appropriate dilutions of the sera. The intra-and interassay coefficients of variation were below 8%. Serum concentrations of CA-125 exceeding 65U/ml were defined as elevated.

RESULTS

Patients

Clinical data of all treated patients are recorded in Table 1, while data from the untreated group are presented in Table 2. At time of primary operation most patients had ovarian cancer stage III or IV according to FIGO classification [11].

The patients' ages varied between 33 and 85 years (mean: 56, median 57 years). The timespan between primary operation and relapse were between 5 and 98 months (mean 32 months, median 19 months). Duration of Decapeptyl administration varied between 1 and 21 months (mean 6.9 months, median 4 months).

By January 1988 six of the 22 treated patients died of progressive disease. Three of these patients presented with severe ascites and pleural effusions as well as with ileus and uremia at initiation of therapy and died within 1 to 3 months. The fourth patient (no. 14) had extensive liver metastases and died 4 months after initiation of Decapeptyl treatment. The other two patients died after 12 and 13 months of treatment respectively. One patient suffered from a stroke and died shortly thereafter.

Treatment was discontinued in three patients. The first refused any further medical treatment. The second developed axillary lymph node metastases after 3 months of treatment, which were expected to be caused by progression of the ovarian cancer. However CA-125 levels remained stable and clinical examinations did not reveal any further abdominal tumor growth. With a progression of lymph node enlargement within 9 months a secondary breast cancer was diagnosed. A parallel rise of the tumor-marker CA 15-3 could be demonstrated by the retrospective analysis of the frozen serum samples (Fig. 1) [12]. In the third patient an increase of CA-125 serum levels associated with the development of intraabdominal tumor has been detected 13 months after primary operation. In that patient we started Decapeptyl administration in combination with oral contraceptives containing 0.25mg levonorgestrel and 0.05mg ethinylestradol (Neogynon 21, Schering AG, Berlin, FRG). During this treatment a decrease of CA-125 was observed and no further growth of the tumors during the next year

Table 1. Clinical data of 19 patients with advanced ovarian cancer. Listed are: initials of patients (init), age at first treatment for ovarian cancer (age), date of first operation (first OP), histological classification (hist) and stage of disease according to FIGO classification (stage), time of secondary surgery (second OP), time of initiation of Decapeptyl administration (Decapep), interval between first operation and initiation of Decapeptyl treatment (Interval I OP-Deca), CA-125 serum levels at start of Decapeptyl administration (CA-125 I), time of death (+), duration of Decapeptyl treatment in months (duration Deca), survival until January 1988 (survival) and last CA-125 serum concentration (CA-125 II).

No.	Init	Age Years	First OP	Hist	Stage	Second OP	Decapep	Interval I OP-Deca	CA-125 I U/ml	+	Duration Deca	Survival Months	CA-125 II U/ml
1	GE	33	02/06/82	s	III	04/22/85	02/16/86	38	70	—	20	68	220
2	HR	35	01/05/78	s	III	08/08/83	03/13/86	98	175	—	21	119	530
3	TE	56	07/12/84	s	IV	02/13/86	03/19/86	20	417	04/25/86		21	-
4	SB	52	10/13/84	s	III	04/22/86	05/05/86	19	412	07/16/86	2	21	4.400
5	ND	69	09/19/85	s	IV	04/16/86	06/11/86	9	65	06/19/87	12	21	7.400
6	GI	54	11/07/85	s	III	03/14/86	08/29/86	9	2.120	12/05/86	3	13	-
7	BT	57	07/06/83	s	III	01/22/85	10/06/86	39	750	08/25/87	13	49	4.500
8	HM	58	11/03/82	s	III	08/30/83	10/30/86	47	188	—	13	60	250
9	RR	44	09/02/83	s	III	05/10/84	11/10/86	38	80	—	13	51	660
10	GM	60	08/29/85	s	III	01/20/87	02/04/87	18	177	—	10	28	8.650 +++
11	BR	51	02/16/86	s	III	07/09/86	03/25/87	13	92	—	9	22	83 +++
12	SK	65	02/01/86	s	IV	06/16/87	03/25/87	16	485	—	9	22	399
13	SB	64	08/04/79	s	III	01/15/87	06/01/87	94	25	—	6	100	25
14	HA	50	07/30/86	s	III	01/19/87	06/25/87	11	2.700	10/16/87	4	15	5.600
15	SL	64	02/17/86	s	III	06/30/87	07/20/87	17	25	—	5	22	25
16	WI	56	07/26/82	s	III	01/16/87	08/20/87	61	781	—	4	65	385 +++
17	HM	52	01/31/84	s	III	03/12/85	08/27/87	43	127	—	4	47	406 +++
18	LL	59	12/15/82	s	III	01/19/87	09/19/87	57	244	—	3	60	348 +++
19	LW	65	04/21/87	s	III	—	09/25/87	5	30	—		8	30
20	HE	85	09/11/86	s	I	—	10/15/87	13	33	12/01/87		14	40
21	WI	47	12/08/84	s	III	12/07/84	12/07/87	36	366	—	1	37	300
22	GE	59	10/14/86	s	III	05/06/87	12/29/87	14	123	—	1	15	157 +++

+++ = patient received oral contraceptives additionally.

Table 2. Clinical data of 11 patients with advanced ovarian cancer. Listed are: initials of patients (init), age at first treatment for ovarian cancer (age), date of first operation (first OP), histological classification (hist) and stage of disease according to FIGO classification (stage), time of secondary surgery or diagnosis of relapse (relapse), interval between first operation and relapse (interval), CA-125 serum levels at time of diagnosis of relapse (CA-125 I), time of death (+), survival after diagnosis of relapse in months (survival overall), survival after diagnosis of relapse (survival relapse) and last CA-125 serum concentration (CA-125 II).

No.	Init	Age Years	First OP	Hist	Stage	Relapse	Interval	CA-125 I U/ml	+	Survival Overall	Survival Relapse	CA-125 II U/ml
1	BM	77	04/04/86	s	III	—	—	490	10/01/87	6	—	1.960
2	SA	59	09/13/85	s	III	04/14/86	7	80	12/09/86	15	8	15.000
3	SI	65	12/21/85	s	III	04/21/86	4	110	10/13/86	10	6	1.220
4	EM	62	06/24/85	s	III	11/25/85	5	43	05/03/86	11	6	3.900
5	WI	56	04/01/86	s	III	08/22/86	7	102	03/15/87	14	7	8.300
6	PB	46	01/31/85	s	III	04/24/86	15	72	09/26/86	20	5	17.200
7	KA	68	05/02/83	s	III	05/12/86	36	83	12/14/86	43	7	406
8	GS	61	07/21/83	s	III	01/28/86	30	700	07/09/86	36	6	1.830
9	RE	73	10/06/86	s	IV	—	—	300	06/13/87	8	—	5.800
10	AB	45	03/17/82	s	III	12/17/85	45	310	10/07/86	55	10	4.900
11	OM	39	04/12/84	s	III	02/22/86	24	640	06/13/86	28	4	4.550

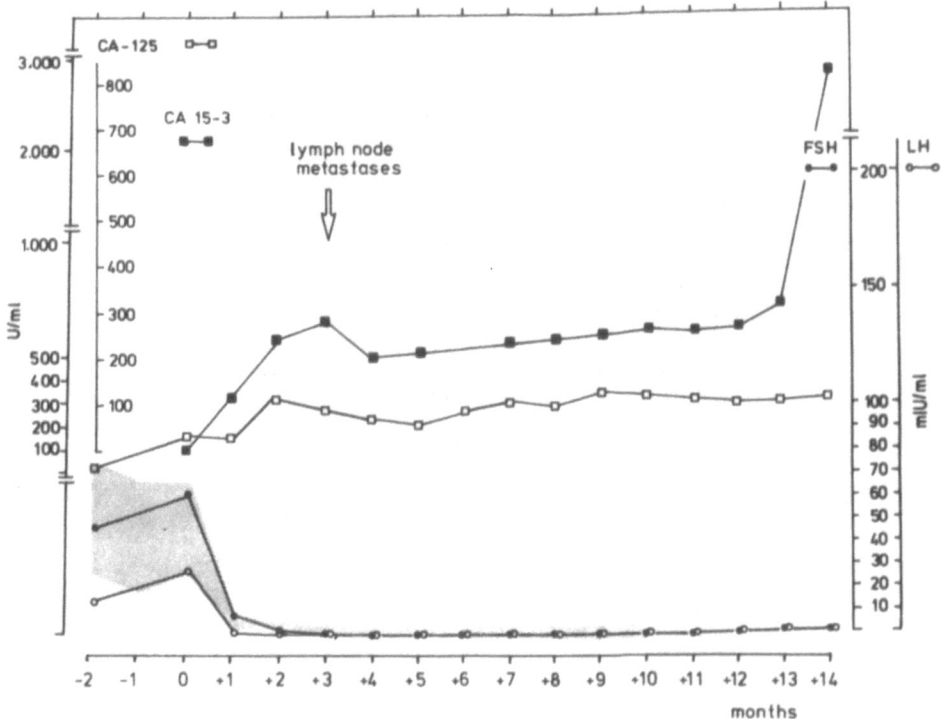

FIGURE 1 Time courses of CA-125, CA 15-3, FSH and LH in patient no 8 (according to Table 1). Time 0 delineates the start of Decapeptyl administration. (Shaded area = range of the gonadotropin levels in treated patients)

(Fig. 2). Therefore she was operated once again in January 1988 using the REGAJ-procedure as described elsewhere [13]. All visible and detectable tumor was removed and the patient is at that point of time without any further treatment.

All 11 patients of the untreated group died between 3 and 11 months after first elevated CA-125 level (Table 2).

FSH and LH levels

In all patients LH and FSH serum levels were elevated before Decapeptyl treatment. In all but one patient the gonadotropin levels decreased after the first injection. While LH levels declined below the detection limit of the assay, FSH levels declined similarly but remained detectable. In two patients the suppression of FSH and LH levels could not be sustained.

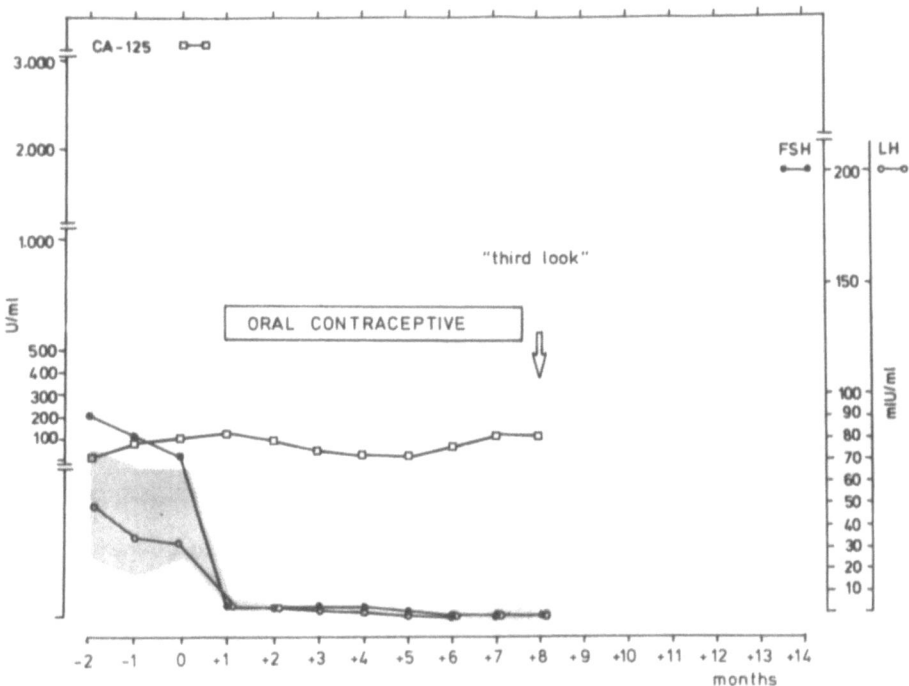

FIGURE 2 Time courses of CA-125, FSH and LH in patient no 11
(according to Table 1). Time 0 delineates the start of
Decapeptyl administration. (Shaded Area = range of the
gonadotropin levels in treated patients)

Therefore the time intervals between Decapeptyl injections were
shortened to 14 days. In the first patient a decline of the LH
and FSH levels within 4 weeks was observed, but after 6 weeks
another increase of the gonadotropins occurred. FSH and levels
remained elevated for 12 weeks and declined without any change
of treatment when she was admitted to the hospital shortly
before she died (Fig. 3).

In the second patient FSH and LH levels increased again
after 8 weeks of Decapeptyl administration. The GnRH-test
revealed an increase of FSH after GnRH injection. Therefore we
decided to shorten the injection intervals. During the next
months FSH levels remained elevated and only a slight reduction
could be noticed (Fig. 4). This patient developed liver
metastases 3 months later, but is without physical complaints
in January 1988.

Six of 7 patients did not respond to the injection of
GnRH with detectable increases of FSH and LH.

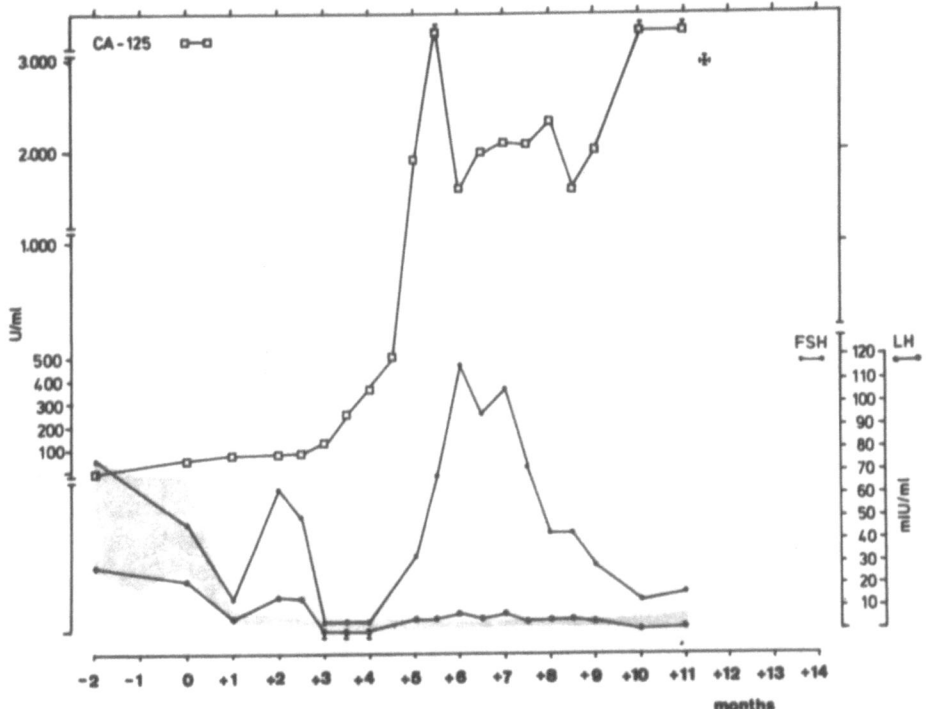

FIGURE 3 Time courses of CA-125, FSH and LH in patient no 5
according to Table 1). Time 0 delineates the start of
Decapeptyl administration. (Shaded area = range of the
gonadotropin levels in treated patients)

In patient no. 10, where FSH and LH levels remained
elevated, the GnRH-test 4 months after initiation of treatment
did not change gonadotropin levels after the injection of GnRH
(Figs. 5 and 6). Therefore we decided to add oral
contraceptives of the combination type. From thereon a
decrease of FSH and LH was documented and the response to GnRH
was completely blocked. From that point of time we started to
administer oral contraceptives together with the Decapeptyl
treatment in a randomized study designed to further reduce the
FSH levels. In all 5 patients treated so far, we observed a
decline of FSH levels to below the lower detected range of the
FSH assay.

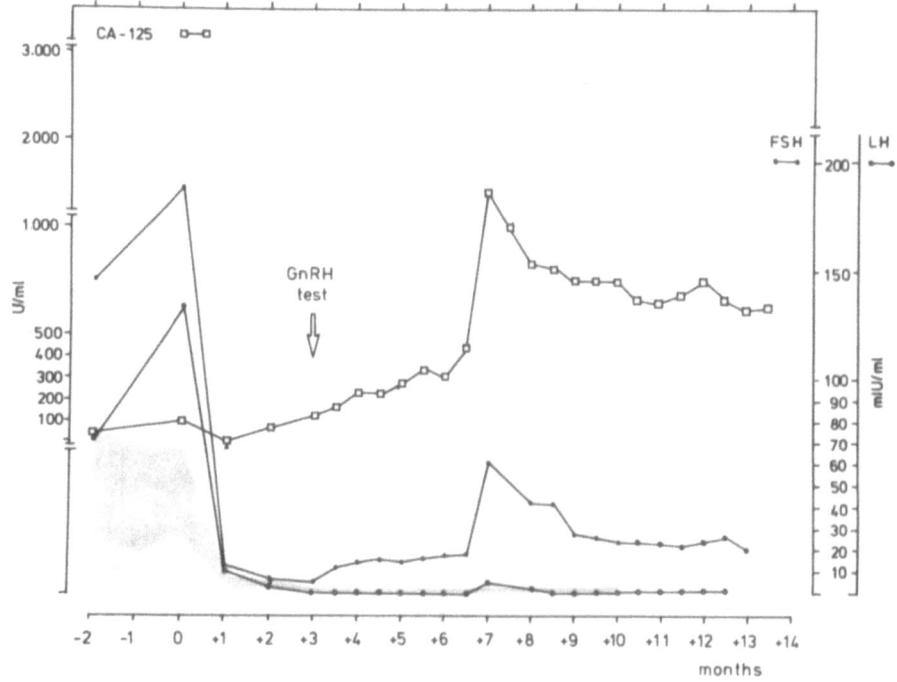

FIGURE 4 Time courses of CA-125, FSH and LH in patient no 9 (according to Table 1). Time 0 delineates the start of Decapeptyl administration. (Shaded area = range of the gonadotropin levels in treated patients)

CA-125 serum levels

In the untreated group the CA-125 concentrations increased rapidly within a few months. During treatment, different patterns of CA-125 serum levels became apparent. Those patients who died shortly after initiation of Decapeptyl administration had comparable changes of the CA-125 serum levels as did the untreated group.

In all other patients treated, although there was a tendency to increase, a considerably slower rate of increase was observed (Figs. 7 and 8).

In two patients the stable course was interrupted by phases of massive increase, when further progression of disease was diagnosed. In one patient CA-125 levels slowly declined but then rapidly increased to a concentrations of 8.650 U/ml. The patient had liver metastases at the initiation of

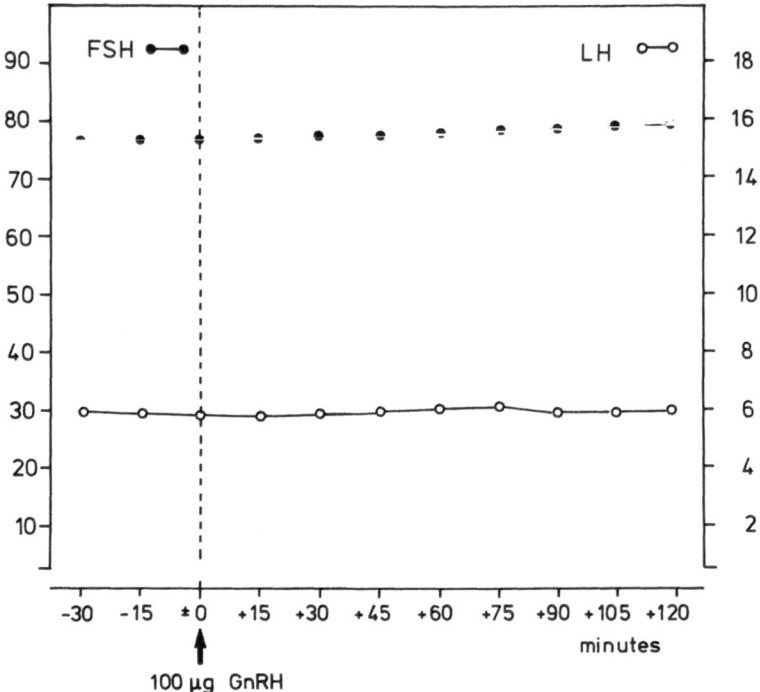

FIGURE 5   FSH and LH serum concentrations during GnRH
          challenge test in patient no 10

Decapeptyl administration, however no remarkable progression
has been observed clinically during that increase so far.   In
one patient a steady decline of CA-125 has now been observed
for more than 4 months.   The recorded liver metastases appear
to be shrinking according to the ultrasound examinations (Fig.
9).

DISCUSSION

In this study we tested the hypothesis that production and
secretion of CA-125 in ovarian cancer is influenced by
pituitary gonadotropins.   Pituitary gonadotropin secretion was
suppressed by the long acting LHRH analogue Decapeptyl and more
recently with the addition of oral contraceptives.
    The results obtained support that hypothesis.   This is
based on the observation that the increase of CA-125 levels was
slower in patients where gonadotropin levels were suppressed

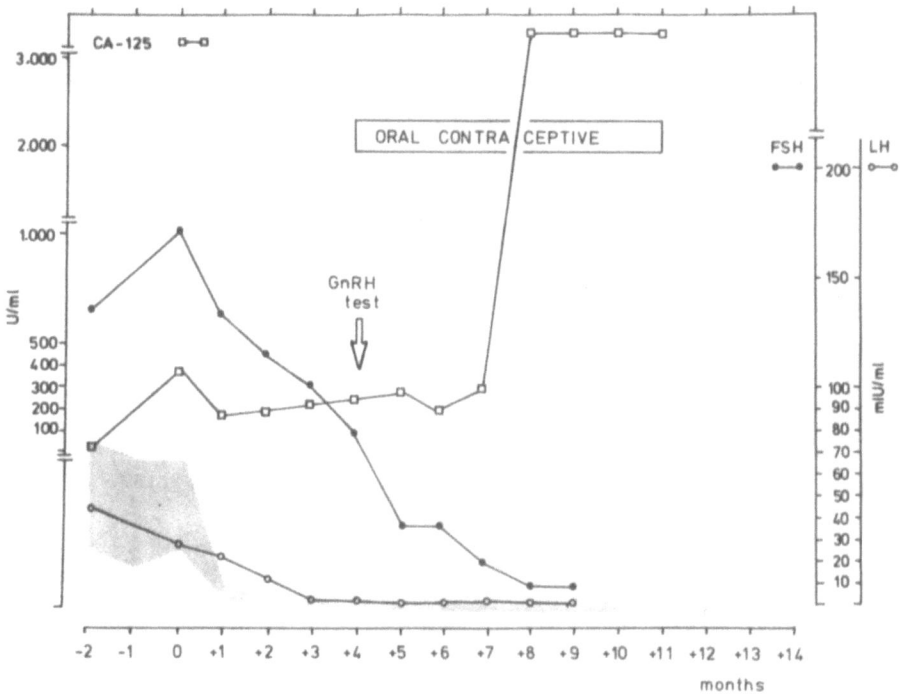

FIGURE 6 Time courses of CA-125, FSH and LH in patient no 10 (according to Table 1). Time 0 delineates the start of Decapeptyl administration. (Shaded area = range of the gonadotropin levels in treated patients). Note massive increase of CA-125 8 months after initiation of treatment

than in those who remained untreated or in whom gonadotropins could not be influenced. The parallel stabilization of disease in 12 of the 19 patients for periods up to 20 months further supports that contention. Whether the addition of hormonal oral contraceptives further improve the course of disease can not be decided yet. Despite the fact that only under that approach in two patients a fall in CA-125 levels was observed, in one patient with liver metastases a dramatic increase of CA-125 appeared after 4 months of the combined modality. However the expected further decline of FSH levels has been demonstrated in all patients treated so far [14].

The time course of CA-125 serum levels has been used as an indirect indicator of the effect of GnRH agonist administration on ovarian cancer. That seemed justified since it had been shown that rising CA-125 serum concentrations are a

181

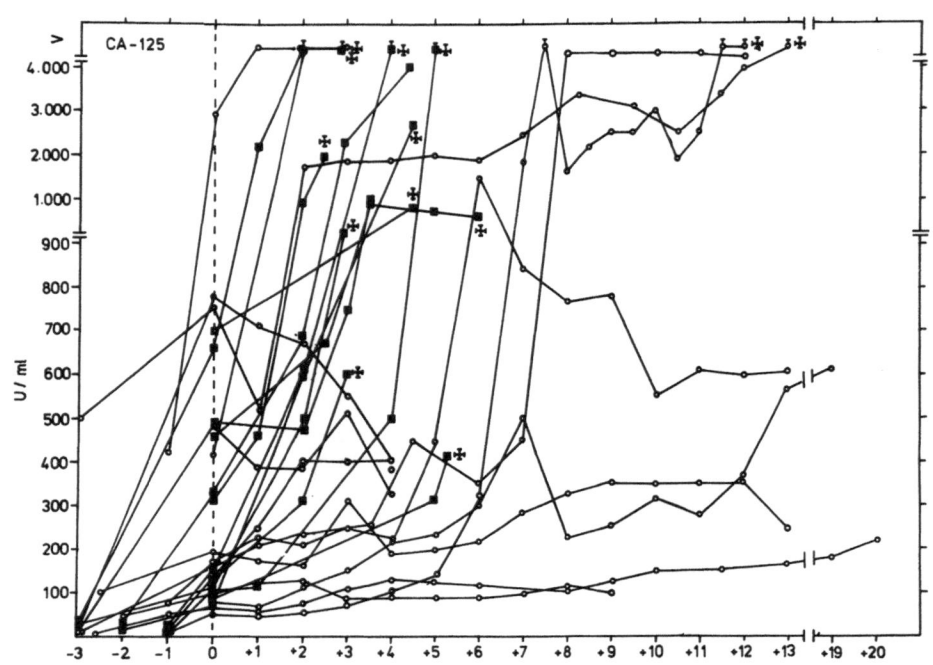

FIGURE 7 CA-125 serum concentrations of all patients. Data
        are normalized to the start of Decapeptyl administration
        for the treated group (0) and for the time of diagnosis of
        recurrence for the untreated group (■)

reliable predictor of progressive tumor growth, in which the
slope of increase Binding sites for GnRH have been demonstrated
in ovarian cancer cells [21]. Nevertheless the observation
that the mirrors the proliferative activity of neoplastic
tissue [5, 6, 15].
      The probability of survival under Decapeptyl
administration is shown in Figure 10 according to the
statistical analysis proposed by Kaplan and Meier [16].
However, we stress that these effects of Decapeptyl
administration and the survival curves have to be interpreted
with utmost caution since patients participating in this study
were not allocated to treated and untreated groups. For this
reason we abstained deliberately from any further rigorous
statistical analysis [17]. The observed effects could be
explained by a direct action of Decapeptyl on ovarian cancerous
tissue or by suppression of pituitary gonadotropin secretion
[18-20].

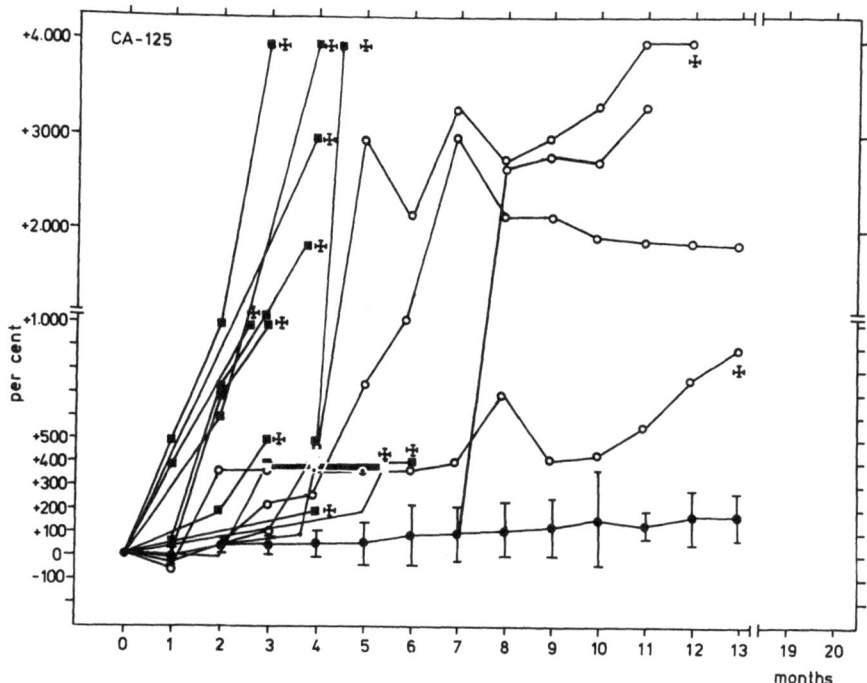

FIGURE 8   Changing levels of the CA-125 serum concentrations
of all patients expressed as percentages of the level at
time 0. The course of 11 patients treated with Decapeptyl
are depicted as mean and standard deviations (⌸). The
CA-125 courses of four patients deviated to a great extent
from the others and are depicted individually (0). Data
are normalized to the start of Decapeptyl administration
for the treated group and for the time of diagnosis of
recurrence for the untreated group (■)

     Binding sites for GnRH have been demonstrated in ovarian
cancer cells [12], Nevertheless the observation that the
gonadotropin levels increased parallel with progressions of
disease although Decapeptyl administration was continued or
even increased would favor the hypothesis that gonadotropins
play a critical role in ovarian cancer and that the effect of
the analogue is mediated by the reduction of circulating
pituitary gonadotropins. Receptors for LH and FSH on ovarian
cancer cells have been described, as well as the enhanced
growth and proliferation of ovarian cancer cells in culture
when FSH was added to the media [22-24].

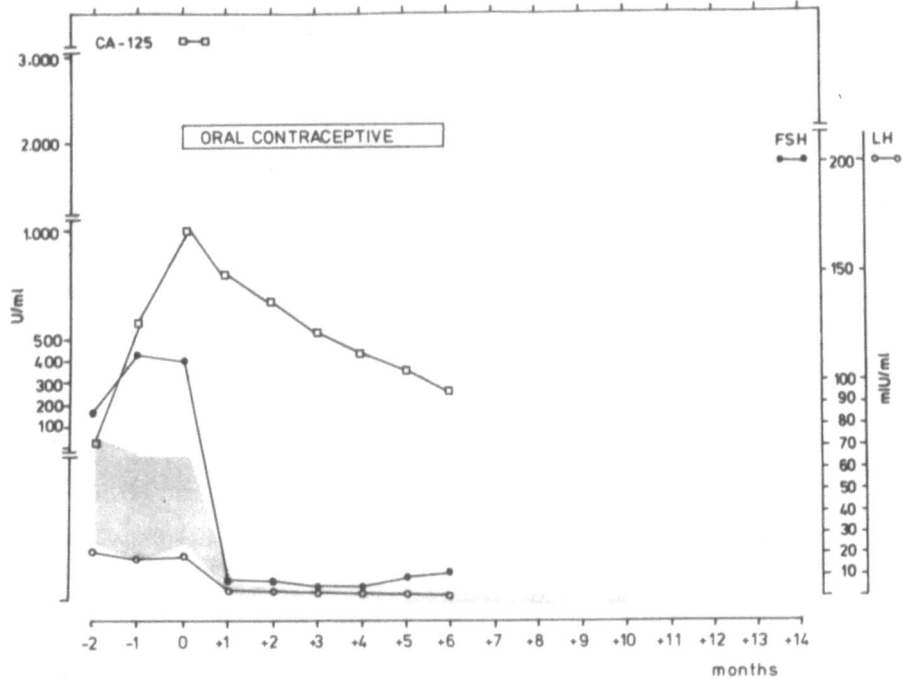

FIGURE 9 Time courses of CA-125, FSH and LH in patient no 16
(according to Table 1). Time 0 delineates the start of
Decapeptyl and oral contraceptive administration. (Shaded
area = range of the gonadotropin levels in treated
patients)

        In addition our data suggest that the regulation of FSH
and LH secretion may escape from controlling mechanisms during
the course of ovarian cancer. The increase of FSH and LH
levels which could not be reduced during therapy or by
shortening of the time interval between injections is not
readily explained and currently under investigation.
        The classical experiments by Biskind and Biskind
demonstrated that the continuous stimulation of rat ovarian
tissue by gonadotropins leads to cancerous changes in the
ovaries [25, 26]. Further exphasis was put on that observation
by the demonstration of Marchant that after hypophysectomy of
the rats no tumours appeared [27].

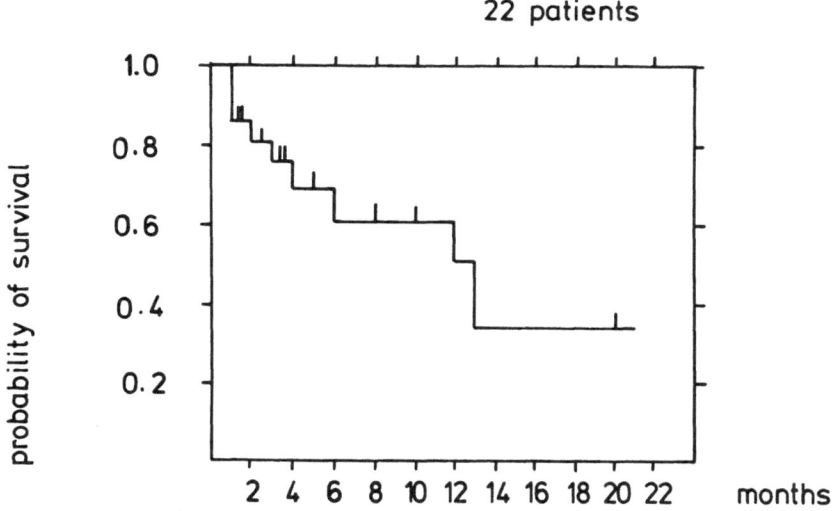

FIGURE 10   Probability of survival for 22 ovarian cancer
     patients during Decapeptyl treatment

        Unfortunately these experiments have not achieved
wide-spread attention and the concept of ovarian cancer as a
hormone dependent neoplastic disease has not been
systematically explored [28, 29]. The development of GnRH
agonists has made it possible to obtain a specific, reversible,
functional hypophysectomy. That should allow us to reevaluate
the role, if any of gonadotropins in the course of ovarian
cancer [30].
        The results obtained so far, although preliminary, are
promising and may provide a point of departure for further
investigation.

REFERENCES

1.   Bast, RC, Feeney, M, Lazarus, H, Nadler, LM, Colvin, RB,
and Knapp, RC (1981). Reactivity of a monoclonal antibody with
human ovarian carcinoma. J Clin Invest, 68, 1331
2.   Kabawat, SE, Bast, RC, Welch, WR, Knapp, RC and Colvin RB
(1983). Immunopathologic characterization of a monoclonal
antibody that recognizes common surface antigens of human
ovarian tumors of serous, endometrioid, and clear types. Am J
Clin Path, 79, 98

3.   Kabawat, SE, Bast, RC, Bhan, AK, Welch, WR, Knapp, RC and
Colvin, RB (1983). Tissue distribution of a
coelomic-epthelium- related antigen recoginzed by the
monoclonal antibody OC 125. Int J Gynecol Pathol, 2, 275
4.   Bast, RC, Klug, TL, St John, E, Jenison, E, Niloff, JM,
Lazarus, H, Berkowitz, RS, Leavitt, T, Griffiths, T, Parker, L,
Zurawski, VR and Knapp, RC (1983). A radioimmunoassay using a
monoclonal antibody to monitor the course of epithelial ovarian
cancer. N Engl J Med, 309, 883
5   Jäger, W, Wildt, L, Braun, P, and Leyendecker, G (1986).
Serumkonzentrationsbestimmungen bei Patientinnen mit
Ovarialkarzinom. In: Wüst, G (ed.) "Tumormarker, aktuelle
Aspekte und klinische Relevanz". p.158. (Darmstadt:
Steinkopff-Verlag)
6.   Bast, RC, Klug, TL, Schaetzl, E, Lavin, P, Niloff, JM,
Greber, TF, Zurawski, VR and Knapp, RC (1984). Monitoring
human ovarian carcinoma with a combination of CA 125, CA 19-9,
and carcinoembryonic antigen. Am J Obstet Gynecol, 149, 553
7.   Jäger, W, Diedrich, K and Wildt, L (1987). Elevated
levels of CA-125 in serum of patients suffering from ovarian
hyperstimulation syndrome. Fertil Steril, 48, 675
8.   Jäger, W, Meier, C, and Wildt, L (1987). Physiological
implication of CA-125 during follicular development and
luteinization? Program of 15th Annual Meeting of the
International Society for Oncodevelopmental Biology and
Medicine, Quebec, August 30 - September 3, 1987, p.86
9.   Jäger, W, Adam, R, Wildt, L and Lang, N (1989). CA-125
serum determination as guideline for timing of second-look
operations and second-line treatment in ovarian cancer
patients. Arch Gynecol, in press
10.   Happ, J, Schultheisis, H, Jacobi, GH, Wenderoth, UK,
Buttenschön, K, Miesel, K, Spahn, and Hör, G (1987).
Pharmacodynamics, pharmacokinetics and bioavailability of the
prolonged LH-RH agonist Decapeptyl-SR. In: Klijn, JGM (ed.)
"Hormonal Manipulation of Cancer, Peptides, Growth Factors, and
New (Anti) Steroidal Agents". p.249. (New York, Raven Press)
11.   FIGO (1971): International federation of gynecology and
obstetrics. Classification and staging of malignant tumours in
the female pelvis. Acta Obstet Gynecol Scand, 50, 1
12.   Jäger, W, Wildt, L, and Leyendecker, G (1986). CA 15-3
and CEA serum concentrations in breast cancer patients. In:
Greten H, Klapdor, R (ed.) "Clinical relevance of new
monoclonal antibodies". p.167. (Stuttgart: Thieme Verlag)
13.   Jäger, W, Lang, N, Feister, N and Wolf, F (1987).
Resection guided by antibodies (iodinized) - REGAJ - a surgical
procedure to detect minor residues of ovarian cancer. J Tumor
Marker Oncol, 2, 64
14.   Lincoln, DW, Fraser, HM, Lincoln, GA, Martin, GB and
McNeilly AS (1985). Hypothalamic pulse generators. Rec Prog
Horm Res, 41, 369

15.   Bast, RC, and Knapp, RC (1985). Use of the CA 125 antigen in diagnosis and monitoring of ovarian carcinoma. Eur J Obstet Gynecol Biol, 19, 345

16.   Kaplan, EL and Meier, P (1958). Non-parametric estimation from incomplete observation. J Am Stat Assoc, 53, 457

17.   Zelen M (1982). Strategy and alternative randomized designs in cancer clinical trials. Cancer Treat Rep, 66, 1095

18.   Schally, AV, Comaru-Schally, AM and Redding, TW (1984). Antitumor effects of analogs of hypothalamic hormones in endocrine-dependent cancers. Proc Soc Exp Biol Med, 175, 259

19.   Cutler, GB, Hoffman, AR, Swerdloff, RS, Santen, RJ, Meldrum DR and Comite, F (1985). Therapeutic applications of luteinizing-hormone-releasing hormone and analogs. Ann Int Med, 102, 643

20.   Conn, PM (1986). The molecular basis of gonadotropin-releasing hormone action. Endocr Rev, 7, 3

21.   Emons, G, Brack, C, Sturm, R, Ball, P and Oberheuser, F (1986). GnRH-binding-sites in human epithelial ovarian carcinoma. Eur J Cancer Clin Oncol, 22, 745

22.   Simon, WE, Albrecht, M, Hänsel, M, Dietel, M and Hölzel, F (1983). Cell lines derived from humn ovarian carcinomas: growth stimulation by gonadotropic and steroid hormones. J Natl Cancer Inst, 70, 839

23.   Rajaniemi, H, Kauppila, A, Rönnberg, L, Selander K and Pystynen, P (1981). LH(hCG) receptor in benign and malignant tumors of human ovary. Acta Obstet Gynecol Scand (Suppl), 101, 83

24.   Bergquist, A, Kullander, S and Thorell, J (1981). A study of oestrogen and progesterone cytosol receptor concentration in benign and malignant ovarian tumours treated with medroxyprogesterone. Acta Obstet Gynecol Scand (Suppl), 101, 75

25.   Biskind, MS and Biskind, GS (1944). Development of tumors in the rat ovary after transplantation into the spleen. Proc Soc Exp Biol Med, 55, 176

26.   Biskind, GR and Biskind, MS (1949). Experimental ovarian tumors in rats. Am J Clin Pathol, 19, 501

27.   Marchant, J (1961). The effect of hypophysectomy on the development of ovarian tumours in mice treated with dimethylbenzanthracene. Brit J Cancer, 15, 821

28.   Cramer, DW, Hutchinson, GB, Welch, WR, Scully, RE and Ryan, KJ (1983). Determinants of ovarian cancer risk. I. Reproductive experiences and family history. J Natl Cancer Inst, 71, 711

29.   Cramer, DW and Welch, WR (1983). Determinants of ovarian cancer risk. II. Inferrences regarding pathogenesis. J Natl Cancer Inst, 71, 717

30.   Bamford, PN and Steele, SJ (1982). Uterine and ovarian carcinoma in a patient receiving gonadotrophin therapy. Case report. Brit J Obstet Gynecol, 89, 962

17
PARTIAL TUMOR REMISSION IN RECURRENT LOW MALIGNANT STROMAL ENDOMETRIOSIS FOLLOWING GnRH AGONIST TREATMENT

TH. BREMEN, S. WAIBEL, G. BENDER, P. HEUSCHEN
and **G. LEYENDECKER**
Department of Obstetrics and Gynecology, Städtische Klinikum,
Grafenstrasse 9, D-6100 Darmstadt, FRG

INTRODUCTION

Hypogonadism caused by the administration of GnRH agonists is of special interest for the treatment of such potentially hormone sensitive tumors as breast cancer [1, 2] and hormone producing ovarian neoplasms [3]. The endometrial stromal cell has been shown to be sensitive to estrogen and progesterone stimulation [4, 5] and is proposed to be the origin of the endometrial stromal sarcoma [6, 7]. Estrogen producing neoplasms such as ovarian granulosa cell tumors or thecomas, polycystic ovarian disease and long term treatment with estrogens in women with gonadal dysgenesis (Turner's syndrome) are associated with a higher risk of developing endometrial stromal sarcomas [8]. It has been reported that the endometrial stromal cell contains cytoplasmic estrogen and progesterone receptors [9, 10].
     Our communication reports a partial tumor remission of a low malignant stromal endometriosis after therapy with a gonadotropin releasing hormone agonist. The results suggest that treatment with GnRH agonists amy be a useful alternative in the therapy of hormone sensitive tumors.

CASE REPORT

A 45-years old woman was admitted to our clinic for the evaluation of a pelvic tumor and multiple suspicious areas in a lung radiograph. A vaginal hysterectomy had been performed three years before because of abnormal bleeding and myomata uteri. Already at this time histological examination of the uterus showed a low malignant stromal endometriosis. No further treatment was started.
     Now gynecological ultrasound and computer tomography showed a 5.5cm tumor consisting of multiple cysts and solid parts. The iliacal and paraaortal lymph nodes were reported to be not enlarged. Laparotomy revealed an endometriosis-like tumor extending from the left pelvic side wall. Intraoperative histological examination could not prove a malignant disease. The

omentum was removed because of multiple adhesions.
Histological examination revealed an endometriosis of the
left ovary. In the omentum multiple metastatic nodes of a low
malignant stromal endometriosis were found. The mitotic index
(number of mitosis per high power field as counted from ten
representative areas) was less than 1.0. Punch biopsies of the
suspicious lung areas showed tumor cells again corresponding to a
low malignant stromal endometriosis.
After surgical treatment the patient was given a regimen of
monhly intramuscular injections of a preparation of micro-capsules
of [D-Trp^6]LHRH (Decapeptyl SR, Ferring Comp., Kiel, FRG).
Serum estradiol and progesterone declined to concentrations of the
early follicular phase during the first month of therapy. The
radiological diameter of the lung metastases was taken as a marker
to control therapy.
X-ray of the chest showed a clearly diminishing size of the
lung metastases four months after the onset of therapy. The
patient has now been under therapy for 11 months. Periodic
examinations including chest radiographs have demonstrated no
evidence of tumor progression.

DISCUSSION

The low malignant stromal endometriosis is a very well
differentiated type of the endometrial stromal sarcoma which
differs from the latter histologically in the very low mitotic
index of the tumor cell [11, 12].
Clinically there is a significant difference in the very
protracted interval between initial treatment and the diagnosis of
recurrence which in low malignant stromal endometriosis is
reported to be as long as 25 years even in FIGO stage I [13].
The very high recurrence rates of 56% in these early stages
of tumor disease [12] make it necessary to establish new methods
of therapy in these cases. Postoperative radiation might be of
benefit to prevent the recurrences in the pelvis [12]. Systematic
cytotoxic chemotherapy results in only 17% of patients with
recurrent stromal endometriosis in partial or complete tumor
remission [12].
Soper et al. [10] reported that about one third of uterine
sarcomas contain high levels of cytoplasmic estrogen or
progesterone receptor concentrations. Baker [9] published on
three cases of low malignant stromal endometriosis with high
concentrations of estrogen and progesterone receptors.
Treatment of recurrent low malignant stromal endometriosis
by long acting synthetic progestins has been reported several
times [9, 12, 14]. Pellili [14] has shown a tumor remission of
lung metastases by weekly intramuscular injections of medroxyprogesterone acetate. Baker [9] demonstrated a case of
postoperative therapy with 160mg of megestrol acetate after
extensive debulking surgery of a progredient stromal
endometriosis. Piver [12] reported a series of 13 patients who

received megestrol, medroxyprogesterone acetate and hydroxypro-
gesterone caproate because of a recurrent stromal endometriosis.
The response rates were about 46% and continued up to 104 months.
     As far as we know our report is the first to describe a
partial tumor remission of a recurrent low malignant stromal
endometriosis after the therapy with a GnRH analog. Recently two
papers on a similar therapy of metastasising leiomyomatosis have
been published [15, 16].
     The patient described has now been in remission for 11
months. The results of our paper may show a new effective
approach to the therapy of these rare tumors. The efficacy of the
therapy of recurrent low malignant stromal endometriosis with GnRH
agonists can only be determined finally by the observation of a
larger number of patients for a longer period of time.

REFERENCES

1.   Mathe, H (1986). Phase II trial of D-Trp-6-LHRH in advanced
breast cancer. Presented at the International symposium on
"Hormonal manipulation of cancer: Peptides, growth factors and new
(anti-) steroidal agents". Rotterdam.
2.   Schally, A, Redding, T, and Comaru-Schally, A (1984).
Potential use of analogs of luteinizing hormone releasing hormones
in the treatment of hormone sensitive neoplasms. Cancer Treat
Rep, 60, 281
3.   Kennedy, L. Traub, A, Atkinson, B, and Sheridan, B (1987).
Short term administration of a gonadotropin releasing hormone
analog to a patient with a testosterone secreting ovarian tumor.
J Clin Endocrinol Metab, 4, 1320
4.   Ferenczy, A and Richat, RM (1978). "Female reproductive
systems: Dynamics of scan and electromicroscopy". (Wiley, New
York).
5.   Wienke, EC (1978). Ultrastructure of the human endometrial
stromal cell during the menstrual cycle. Am J Obstet Gynecol,
102, 65
6.   Kudo, R (1973). Ultrastructural study of endometrial
stromal sarcoma or stromal endometriosis. Acta Obstet Gynecol
Japon, 20, 73
7.   Mazun, MT and Agkin, B (1978). Endolymphatic stromal myosis
-unique presentation of an ultrastructured study. Cancer, 42, 2661
8.   Press, MF, and Scully, RE (1985). Endometrial "sarcomas"
complicating ovarian thecoma, polycystic ovarian disease and
estrogen therapy. Gynecol Oncol, 21, 135
9.   Baker, VV, Walton, LA, Fowler, WC and Currie, SC (1984).
Steroid receptors in endolymphatic stromal myosis. Obstet
Gynecol, 63 (Suppl.), 72
10.   Soper, JT, Mc Carthy, K, Hinshaw, W, Creasmann, WT, Mc
Carthy, K and Clarke-Pearson, D (1984). Cytoplasmic estrogen and
progesterone receptor content of uterine sarcomas. Am J Obstet
Gynecol, 150, 342

11.   Kahanpää, KV, Wahlstrom, T, Gröhn, P, Heinonen, E, Nieminen, U, and Widholm, P (1986). Sarcomas of the uterus: a clinico-pathological study of 119 patients. Obstet Gynecol, 67, 417

12.   Piver, M St, Rutledge, FN, Copeland, L, Webster, K, Blumenson, L and Suh, O (1984). Uterine endolymphatic stromal myosis: a collaborative study. Obstet Gynecol, 64, 173

13.   Krieger, PD and Gusberg, SB (1973). Endolymphatic stromal myosis - A grade I endometrial sarcoma. Gynecol Oncol, 1, 299

14.   Pellilli, D (1968). Proliferative stromatosis of the uterus with pulmonary metastases. Remission following treatment with a long acting synthetic progestin: A case report. Obstet Gynecol, 31, 33

15.   Hague, WM, Abdulwahid, NA, Jacobs, HS and Craft, I (1986). Use of LHRH analogue to obtain reversible castration in a patient with a benign metastasing leiomyoma. Brit J Obstet Gynecol, 93, 455

16.   Maheux, R, Samson, Y, Fariel, NR, Parent, JG and Jean, C (1987). Utilization of luteinizing hormone releasing hormone agonist in pulmonary leiomyomatosis. Fertil Steril, 48, 315

18

ENDOCRINE, PHARMACOKINETIC AND CLINICAL EFFECTS OF LHRH ANALOGUE TREATMENT IN PATIENTS WITH MALIGNANT AND BENIGN BREAST DISEASE

J.G.M. KLIJN[1], A.N. VAN GEEL[1], F.H. DE JONG[2] and J. SANDOW[3]
[1]Division of Endocrine Oncology and Department of Surgery,
The Rotterdam Cancer Institute, Rotterdam, The Netherlands
[2]Department of Medicine II and Clinical Endocrinology,
Erasmus University, Rotterdam, The Netherlands
[3]Department of Pharmacology, Hoechst AG, Frankfurt, FRG

INTRODUCTION

Since 1981 it has been apparent that LHRH analogues can be used for suppression of pituitary gonadotropin secretion and for reaching "medical castration" in the treatment of hormone-dependent malignant and benign diseases, especially because of the absence of serious side effects [1-4]. The efficacy of this type of treatment has been established in patients with prostate cancer by a large number of invesigators [1-7] as well as by our group [8-11]. Since our first report in 1982 [12] on the use of LHRH analogues in the treatment of metastatic breast cancer in premenopausal women, the number of studies in this type of patients has been increasing, but results of treatment in patients with mastalgia have not been reported. A number of phase II studies in breast cancer indicate that chronic treatment with LHRH analogues is generally as effective as other common kinds of endocrine therapy in premenopausal breast cancer with respect to response rate, duration of response and survival [12-29]. However, randomized comparative studies have yet to be performed.

As an analogy with complete androgen blockade using combined LHRH agonist and an antiandrogen in the treatment of prostate cancer [5, 11], complete estrogen blockade by means of combined treatment with an LHRH agonist and an antiestrogen might be attractive in the treatment of breast cancer. However, the antiestrogen tamoxifen enhances the stimulatory effect of the LHRH agonist on pituitary function in about half of the patients when the LHRH agonist is administered intranasally before [13-16]. Recently we found that subcutaneous treatment with high doses of the LHRH agonist buserelin (twice daily injections of 1mg) is much more effective than intranasal treatment [16-20]. However, one of the questions to be addressed is whether high dose subcutaneous treatment with an LHRH agonist can prevent the stimulatory effect

of tamoxifen on pituitary-ovarian function in premenopausal
women. Therefore, we have studied the effects of combined
treatment with tamoxifen and high dose buserelin s.c. in a
subgroup of 9 patients with metastatic breast cancer [20]. In
addition, we have investigated the potential clinical benefit,
endocrine effects and pharmacokinetics of treatment with buserelin
implants in 6 patients with mastalgia especially with respect to
the duration of estrogen suppression after application of the last
buserelin implant.

PATIENTS, TREATMENT AND METHODS

Since 1981 we have administered buserelin as a first line
treatment to 46 premenopausal patients with metastatic breast
cancer, using various treatment regimens (Table 1).

Table 1   Treatment regimens and response rate in premenopausal
breast cancer patients

Group	Treatment	CR + PR	No Change	Failure
I A	Buserelin i.n.	4	4	4
I B	Buserelin s.c.	5	1	5
II A	Buserelin i.n. + TAM	3	0	2
II B	Buserelin i.n. + MA	2	1	1
II C	Buserelin s.c. + TAM	4	3	7
Total		18 (39%)	9 (20%)	19 (41%)

CR = complete response, PR = partial response, TAM = Tamoxifen,
MA = megestiol acetate

Twenty-three patients were treated with buserelin (12 and
3x400µg intranasally, 11 with 2x1mg subcutaneously) as single
treatment and 23 received buserelin in combination with tamoxifen
(TAM) or megestrol acetate (MA).
     Six premenopausal patients with mastalgia gave informed
consent to be treated with 2 PLGA 50:50 buserelin implants of
3.3mg s.c. every 4 weeks. One of these patients was also operated
on for primary breast cancer and needed contraception. The
treatment started in the last week of the menstrual cycle. The
duration of treatment was 24 weeks in 4 patients, 12 weeks in one
and 62 weeks with an increasing interval between the implantations
in our first patient.
     Levels of estradiol (E_2), progesterone, LH and FSH in
weekly plasma samples and urinary buserelin levels were measured
by radioimmunoassay [31, 32]. In a number of patients plasma
samples were also collected for buserelin measurements. Tumor
responses were evaluated according UICC criteria.

RESULTS

Clinical effects

Of the 46 premenopausal patients with metastatic breast cancer 18 (39%) showed a objective response and 9 (20%) stabilization of disease, while 19 patients (41%) had progressive tumor growth from the start of treatment.

In the 6 patients with mastalgia this complaint disappeared or decreased, but reccurred when plasma E_2 levels increased after cessation of treatment. Normoprolactinemic galactorrhea, which was present in one patient, did not respond to bromocriptine treatment, and did not disappear during treatment with the buserelin implants in spite of very low plasma E_2 concentrations. One patient refused further treatment after 3 implantations because of the occurrence of severe hot flushes every half hour in the presence of undetectable plasma E2 concentrations.

Endocrine effects

Part of the endocrine effects of these treatment regimens has been described before [12-20]. Most important for the present discussion are the endocrine effects of treatment with subcutaneous injections of high doses of buserelin in combination with 2x20mg tamoxifen and in the patients with mastalgia treated with buserelin implants. All patients became amenorrhoic during chronic treatment in the presence of continuously low plasma progesterone levels. After an initial rise on the first day plasma immunoassayable gonadotropin levels decreased to the lower limit of the normal range within 2-3 weeks and remained low during the treatment period (Fig. 1).

In the group of patients treated with buserelin injecions plus tamoxifen, plasma E_2 concentrations decreased to castrate levels in all patients within 3 weeks with a mean plasma E_2 level of 25 pmol/l [20]. No recurrent peaks of E_2 were observed, in contrast wih the results in half of the patients who were treated with intranasal application of buserelin and a similar dose of tamoxifen.

In the group of patients with mastalgia plasma E_2 levels fell to castrate levels in all patients within 2 weeks and remained low afterwards [20]. All patients experienced hot flushes after 2-3 weeks of treatment. The mean plasma E_2 concentration in this group of patients was significantly (p<0.01) lower than in 100 postmenopausal controls, i.e. 17 vs 34 pmol/l[20]. After stopping treatment with the buserelin implants, suppression of ovarian E_2 secretion continued for 15-20 weeks and amenorrhea persisted for 18 to more than 22 weeks after the last buserelin implantation.

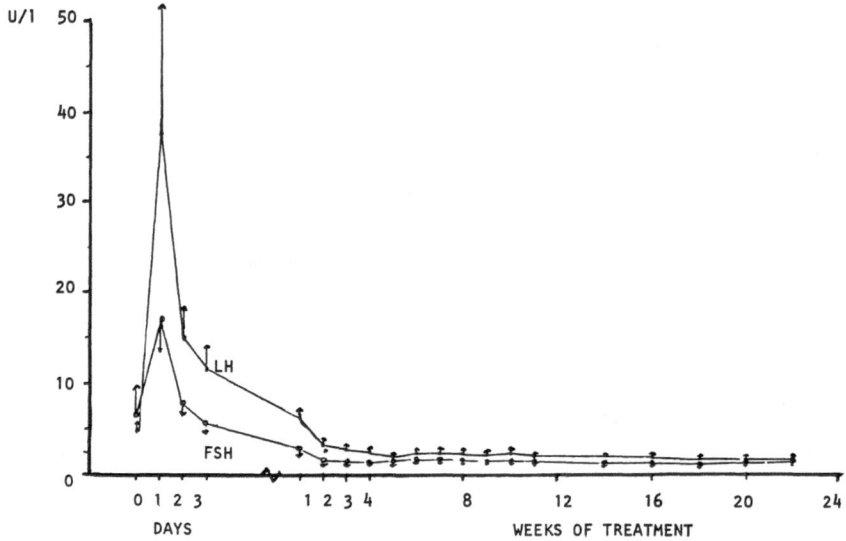

FIGURE 1 Plasma concentrations of LH and FSH in 6 patients
treated with 2x1mg buserelin s.c. plus 2x20mg tamoxifen (mean
± SEM).

Pharmacokinetics of buserelin released from subcutaneous implants

In one patient we measured the rise in plasma and urinary
buserelin levels every hour during the first 6 hours and after 24
hours on the first treatment day. Plasma and urinary peak values
were reached after 5 hours with peak values of 0.87ng/ml in plasma
and 250µg per gram creatinine in the urine. After 24 hours
these values were decreased to 0.28ng/ml and 42µg per gram
creatinine respectively. During the next 4 weeks plasma buserelin
levels remained more or less constant while urinary buserelin
excretion decreased slowly.
        In the whole group of 6 patients mean urinary buserelin
excretion during the first treatment cycle was lower than that
observed during the first three weeks of the next treatment
cycles; no differences were observed between mean urinary
buserelin levels during cycles 2-6 (Fig. 2). Four weeks after the
implantation mean buserelin excretion was equivalent in the first
and all other cycles (about 24µg/g creatinine).

196

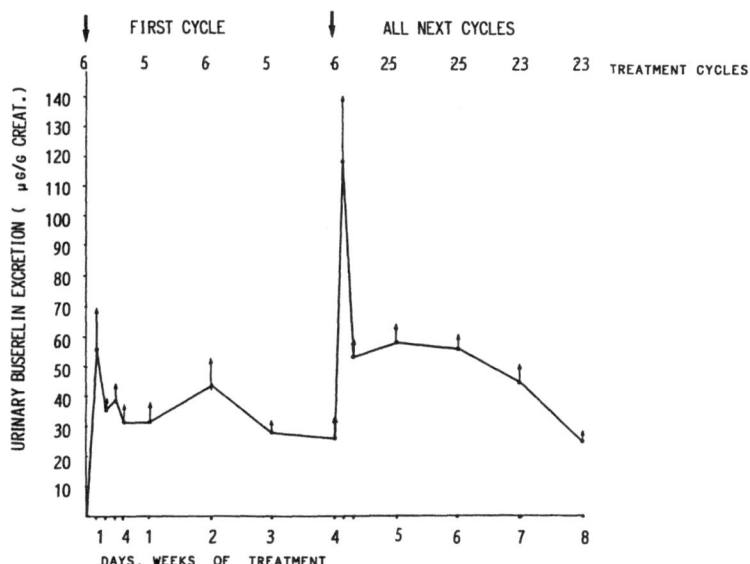

FIGURE 2 Buserelin pharmacokinetics: urinary buserelin
excretion (mean ± SEM) during treatment with PLG 50:50
buserelin implants in 6 patients with mastalgia for 24 weeks.

After the last implantation buserelin excretion remained
relatively high (more than 5µg/g creatinine) during at least 8
weeks followed by a logarithmic decrease to undetectable levels at
17 to more than 20 weeks after the last implantation. In the 4
patients treated with 6 implants of 6.6mg buserelin, a rise of
plasma E_2 levels did not occur before buserelin excretion was
lower than 0.1-0.2µg buserelin/g creatinine.

DISCUSSION AND CONCLUSIONS

In premenopausal metastatic breast cancer chronic LHRH agonist
treatment appears as effective as other common kinds of endocrine
therapy [12-29]. In 7 studies [17, 21, 24, 26-29], on a total of
138 patients, 40% showed an objective response (Table 2).

Table 2 Survey of literature responses of premenopausal breast cancer patients to treatment with LHRH agonists

Author	Ref.	LHRH Agonist	N	CR + PR
1) Klijn et al.	17	Buserelin	23	9 (39%)
2) Nicholson et al.	24	Zoladex	45	14 (31%)
3) Harvey et al.	21	Leuprolide	25	11 (44%)
4) Mathe et al.	26	Tryptorelin	8	3 (38%)
5) Höffken et al.	27	Buserelin	15	7 (47%)
6) Kaufmann et al.	28	Zoladex	12	5 (42%)
7) Wander et al.	29	Zoladex	10	6 (60%)
			138	55 (40%)

Overall objective response rate of ER-positive tumors: 36/70 (51%). Longest duration of response: 5 years.

The overall objective response rate in patients with estradiol receptor positive tumors was 51%, while tumor regression occurred rarely in patients with steroid receptor negative breast tumors. Thus far the longest duration of response is 5 years. However, randomized studies have still to be carried out to prove that LHRH agonist treatment is indeed as effective as other types of endocrine treatment. Tamoxifen can safely be combined with high s.c. doses of LHRH agonist or by implants in order to reach "complete estrogen blockade" [20, 25]. In order to investigate this point in more detail, the EORTC Breast Cancer Cooperative Group is presently conducting a randomized study comparing the effects of treatment with buserelin implants alone versus buserelin implants plus tamoxifen versus tamoxifen alone.
     Treatment with buserelin implants had a clear beneficial effect in our patients with mastalgia. However, this kind of treatment has its limitations, firstly because of long duration of treatment has the potential risk of bone loss, and secondly because of the observed reccurence of complaints when plasma E2 levels rise after cessation of treatment. In our study there was a strong suppression of peripheral E2 levels to 50% below mean postmenopausal plasma concentrations during at least 12 weeks from start of treatment [20]. From an endocrine point of view treatment with buserelin implants every 4-12 weeks is as effective as treatment with 2 daily s.c. injections of 1mg buserelin. Most importantly, it appeared in our study that peripheral concentrations of buserelin which give rise to urinary excretion as low as 0.2µg/g creatinine can continuously suppress pituitary-ovarian function when continuously released from implants.

REFERENCES

1.   Corbin, A (1982). From contraception to cancer: a review of the therapeutic applications of LHRH analogues as antitumour agents. Yale J Biol Med, 55, 27
2.   Furr, BJA and Nicholson, RI (1982). Use of analogues of luteinizing hormone-releasing hormone for the treatment of cancer. J Reprod Fert, 64, 529
3.   Sandow, J (2983). Clinical applications of LHRH and its analogues. Clin Endocrinol, 18, 571
4.   Schally, AV, Redding, TW and Comaru-Schally, AM (1984). Potential use of analogs of luteinizing hormone-releasing hormones in the treatment of hormone-sensitive neoplasms. Cancer Treat Rep, 68, 2819
5.   Labrie, F, Belanger, A, Dupont, A, Emond, J, Lacoursiere, Y and Monfette, G (1984). Combined treatment with LHRH agonist and pure antiandrogen in advanced carcinoma of prostate. Lancet, ii, 1090
6.   Garnick, MB, Glode, LM and the Leuprolide Study Group (1984). Leuprolide versus diethylstilbestrol for metastatic prostate cancer. New Engl J Med, 311, 1281
7.   Parmar, H, Lightman, SL, Allen, L, Philips, RH, Edwards, L and Schally, AV (1985). Randomised controlled study of orchidectomy versus long-acting D-TRP-6-LHRH microcapsules in advanced prostatic carcinoma. Lancet, ii, 1201
8.   De Jong, FH, Schroeder, FH, Lock, MTWT, Debruyne, FMJ, De Voogt, HJ and Klijn, JGM (1987). Effects of long-term treatment with the LHRH-analogue buserelin on the pituitary-testicular axis in men with prostatic carcinoma (PCA). In: Klijn, JGM, Paridaens, R and Foekens, JA (eds.) "Hormonal manipulation of Cancer: Peptides, Growth Factors and New(Anti) Steroidal Agents, EORTC Monograph Series" vol 18, p.195. (New York: Raven Press)
9.   Schroeder, FJ, Lock, TMTW, Chadha, DR, Debruyne, FMJ, Karthausk HFM, de Jong, FH, Klijn, JGM. Matroos. AW and de Voogt, HJ (1987). Metastatic cancer of the prostate managed with buserelin versus buserelin plus cyproterone acetate. J Urol, 137, 912
10.   Klijn, JGM, de Jong, FH, Lamberts, SWJ and Blankenstein, MA (1984). LHRH-agonist treatment in metastatic prostate carcinoma. Eur J Cancer Clin Oncol, 20, 483
11.   Klijn, JGM, De Voogt, HJ, Schroder, F.H. and de Jong, FH (1985). Combined treatment with buserelin and cyproterone acetate in metastic prostate carcinoma. Lancet, 11, 493
12.   Klijn, JGM and de Jong, FH (1982). Treatment with a luteinizing hormone-releasing-hormone analogue (buserelin) in premenopausal patients with metastatic breast cancer. Lancet, i, 1213
13.   Klijn, JGM (1984). Long--term LHRH-agonist treatment in metastatic breast cancer as a single treatment and in combination with other additive endocrine treatment. Med Oncol Tumor Pharmacother, 1, 123

14.   Klijn, JGM and de Jong, FH (1984).   Long-term treatment with the LHRH-agonist buserelin (Hoe 766) for metastatic breast cancer in single and combined drug regimen.   In: Labrie, F, Belanger, A, and Dupont, A (eds.) "LHRH and its Analogues, Basic and Clinical Aspects. p. 425. (Amsterdam: Excerpta Medica)

15.   Klijn, JGM, de Jong, FH, Blankenstein, MA, Docter, R Alexieva-Figusch, J, Blonk-van der Wijst, J and Lamberts, SWJ (1984). Anti-tumor and endocrine effects of chronic LHRH agonist (buserelin) treatment with or without tamoxifen in premenopausal metastatic breast cancer. Breast Cancer Res Treat, 4, 209

16.   Klijn, JGM, De Jong, FH, Lamberts, SWJ and Blankenstein, MA (1985). LHRH-agonist treatment in clinical and experimental human breast cancer. J Steroid Biochem, 23, 867

17.   Klijn, JGM and de Jong, FH (1987).   Long-term LHRH-agonist (buserelin) treatment in metastatic premenopausal breast cancer. In Klijn, JGM, Paridaens, R and Foekens, JA (eds.) "Hormonal Manipulation of Cancer: Peptides, Growth Factors and New (Anti) steroidal Agents, EORTC Monograph Series, Vol 18, p 343. (New York, Raven Press)

18.   Klijn, JGM, Henkelman, MS and Bakker, GH (1987).   Treatment of premenopausal metastatic breast cancer or endometriosis with LHRH-analogues.   In: Englesman, E and de Koning Gans, HJ (eds.) "Proceedings of the Symposium on Endocrine-Related Tumours" p. 160.   (London: The Update Seibert Group Limited)

19.   Klijn, JGM and Foekens, JA (1988).   Long-term peptide hormone treatment with LHRH-agonist in metastatic breast cancer. In: Santen, R (ed.) "Proceedings of the Symposium of Endocrine-Dependent Breast Cancer, Critical Assessment of Recent Advances, 14th International Cancer Congress" August 20-7, Budapest (in press)

20.   Klijn, JGM, van Geel, AN and de Jong, FH (1988).   Endocrine effects of LHRH-agonist (buserelin) implants and of combined treatment of high dose buserelin s.c. with tamoxifen in premenopausal women.   In: Proceedings of the 3rd International Congress on Hormones and Cancer, September 1987, Hamburg (in press)

21.   Harvey, HA, Lipton, A and Max, DT (1987). LHRH agonist treatment of breast cancer: a phase II study in the USA.   In: Klijn, JGM, Paridaens, R and Foekens, JA (eds.) "Hormonal Manipulation of Cancer: Peptides, growth Factors and New (Anti) steroidal Agents".   EORTC Monograph Series, vol 18. (New York: Raven Press)

22.   Manni, A, Santen, R, Harvey, H, Lipton, A and Max, D (1986).   Treatment of breast cancer with gonadotropin releasing hormone. Endocr Rev, 7, 89

23.   Nicholson, RI, Walker, KJ, Turkes, A, Dyas, J, Plowman, PN, Williams, M and Blamey, RW (1985).   Endocrinological and clinical aspects of LHRH action (ICI-118630) in hormone dependent breast cancer. J Steroid Biochem, 23, 843

24.   Nicholson, RI, Walker, KJ, Turkes, A, Dyas, J, Plowman, PN, Williams, M, Elston, CW and Blamey, RW (1987). The British experience with the LHRH-agonist Zoladex (ICI-118630) in the treatment of breast cancer. In: Klijn, JGM, Paridaens, R and Foekens JA (eds.) "Hormonal Manipulation of Cancer: Peptides, Growth Factors and New (Anti) steroidal Agents". EORTC Monograph Series, Vol 18, p. 331. (New York: Raven Press)

25.   Nicholson, RI, Walker, KJ, Walker, RF, Read, GF, Finlay, E, Robertson, J, Blamey, RW and Griffiths, K (1988). Oestrogen deprivation in breast cancer using LHRH agonist and antioestrogens. In: Proceedings of the 3rd Internationl Congress in Hormone and Cancer, September 1987, Hamburg (in press)

26.   Mathe, G, Keiling, R, Vovan, ML, Gastiaburu, J, Prevot, G, Vannetzel, JM, Despax, R, Jasmin, C, Levi, F, Musset, M, Machover, D and Misset, JL (1986). Phase II trial of D-Trp-6-LHRH in advanced breast cancer. Eur J Cancer Clin Oncol, 22, 723

27.   Hoefken, K, Miller, B, Fischer, P, Becker, R, Kurschel, E, Scheulen, ME, Miller, AA, Callis, R and Schmidt, CG (1986). Buserelin in treatment of premenopausal advanced breast cancer. Eur J Cancer Clin Oncol, 22, 746

28.   Kaufman, M (1987). Treatment of advanced breast cancer with a long acting depot preparation of a synthetic GnRH-agonist (Zoladex) in premenopausal patients. Program of 4th EORTC Breast Cancer Working Conference, abstr. F 1.8

29   Wander, HE, Keelberg, UR, Schachner-Wünschmann, E and Nagel, GA (1987). A long-acting depot preparation of a synthetic GnRH agonist (Zoladex) in the treatment of pre- and postmenopausal advanced breast cancer. J Steroid Biochem, 28, (suppl), 104 S, abstract C-017

30   Manni, A and Pearson, OH (1980). Antiestrogen-induced remissions in premenopausal women with Stage IV breast cancer: effects on ovarian function. Cancer Treat Rep, 64, 779

31.   Klijn, JGM, Lamberts, SWJ, deJong, FH, Docter, R, van Dongen, KJ and Birkenhäger, JC (1980). The importance of pituitary tumour size in patients with hyperprolactinaemia in relation to hormonal variables and extrasellar extension of tumour. Clin Endocrinol, 12, 341

32.   Sandow, J, Seidel, HR, Krauss, B and Jerabek-Sandow, G (1987). Pharmacokinetics of LHRH agonists in different delivery systems and the relation to endocrine function. In: Klijn, JGM, Paridaens, R and Foekens, JA (rds.) "Hormonal manipulation of Cancer: Peptides, Growth Factors and New (Anti) Steroidal Agents". EORTC Monograph Series, vol 18, p 203. (New York: Raven Press)

19

LHRH AGONISTS AS ADJUNCTS TO SOMATOSTATIN ANALOGS IN THE TREATMENT OF PANCREATIC CANCER

Ana Maria COMARU-SCHALLY and **Andrew V. SCHALLY**
Endocrine Polypeptide and Cancer Institute, Veterans Administration
Medical Center, and Section of Experimental Medicine,
Department of Medicine, Tulane University School of Medicine,
New Orleans, Louisiana 70146, USA

INTRODUCTION

The incidence of adenocarcinoma of the exocrine pancreas is steadily increasing [1-3]. Approximately 25,000 new cases of pancreatic cancer are diagnosed yearly in the USA where this tumor now ranks as the fourth leading cause of death from malignancies. The vast majority of pancreatic cancers are ductal adenocarcinomas, but other pancreatic carcinomas also occur [1-3]. Histogenetically, more than 90% of these tumors are derived from the pancreatic ducts and thus about 60% are located in the head of the gland [1]. Ductal adenocarcinoma has a very poor prognosis, in part because most patients have advanced disease by the time of diagnosis [1-4]. Early diagnosis and screening for nonendocrine pancreatic cancer is difficult, although the technology for detecting these small tumors is available [1-7]. Delay in detection is mostly due to the fact that early symptoms are usually vague and nonspecific and very often neglected by the patients and missed by the physicians [1, 3, 5, 6]. Thus clinicians should be alert to the problem and look for it in the appropriate setting. Mortality due to carcinomas of the exocrine pancreas is very high and the great majority of patients die within a year from the time of diagnosis [3, 8]. The generally accepted 5-year survival rate is 1-5% in resectable disease [1, 3, 8, 9]. Moreover, many die later of recurrent disease [1, 2].

Current treatments for ductal adenocarcinoma of the pancreas have little effect on its outcome. Surgery at present is the only modality with curative potential but the resectability rate in most series is only about 15 to 20% [3]. Nowadays, pancreatic resection can be performed in some specialized centres with an acceptably low operative mortality and morbidity [1, 2 5]. However, there is no general agreement about whether resection prolongs life because it is difficult to stage tumors preoperatively for proper comparison in controlled trials [5]. Attempts have been made to enhance post-resection survival time by combining radiation therapy with 5-fluorouracil (5-FU) therapy following pancreatic resection [10]. The findings of this study

were that the group treated with combined therapy had a 48%
survival at 2 years versus anticipated 18% survival for
pancreatectomy alone [10]. Unfortunately, only a small percentage
of patients with cancer of the head of the pancreas can be
selected for this adjuvant combined modality therapy and operative
mortality, risk of complications, side effects, quality of life,
and long term survival must be considered with this approach [1,
2]. Early trials with the combination of 5-FU plus radiotherapy
in patients with locally unresectable pancreatic carcinom
demonstrated a median survival of 40 weeks [11]. Median survival
with radiation alone was reported to be 37 months from date of
diagnosis [11]. Chemotherapy with single or multiple agents for
inoperable pancreatic cancer has resulted in only modest
improvement in response rates [1, 3, 8, 12]. High-dose external
beam irradiation in combination with 5-FU or FAMS (5-FU,
adriamycin, mitomycin C, streptozocin) was recommended to palliate
patients with inoperable tumors and those unfit for a major
pancreatic resection [1].
　　　Thus carcinoma of the exocrine pancreas poses a challenge to
physicians. Early diagnosis is difficult, the outlook for cure
remains poor and the death rate continues to approximate the
incidence [1-12]. More research on this disease is needed
including the research for new effective nonsurgical therapy. A
possible new approach to treat this malignancy has been proposed
by our group and is based on chronic administration of hormonal
peptide analogs [13-18].

POSSIBLE HORMONAL DEPENDENCE OF PANCREATIC CANCER

Various findings suggest that it might be possible to develop a
new hormonal therapy for malignant exocrine tumors of the pancreas
based on new somatostatin analogs, alone or in combination with
LHRH analogs [13-18]. Potent analogs of somatostatin were
synthesized by several groups including ours [19-21]. Studies
carried out during the past 14 years have shown that
somatostatin-14, somatostatin-28 and their analogs exert
inhibitory actions on the pancreas as well as on the stomach and
gut [22-29]. These actions include inhibition of the release of
insulin and glucagon from the pancreas and suppression of the
secretion and/or action of gastrin, secretin, cholecystokinin
(CCK), vasoactive intestinal peptide (VIP) and pancreatic
polypeptide [13, 22-29]. Gastrin, CCK, caerulein and secretin
promote the growth of the exocrine pancreas and increase DNA, RNA
and protein content [30-33]. The production of hyperplasia and
hypertrophy of the exocrine pancreas by gastrin, CCK and secretin
is now well established [30-32]. It is likely that these
gastrointestinal (GI) hormones also influence the growth of the
malignant cells of the pancreas and phenotypic transformations
[33-36]. Although tumors of the endocrine pancreas will not be
discussed in this review, it is worth mentioning that somatostatin
and its analogs were effective in inhibiting the synthesis and/or
release of polypeptides from islet-cell tumors [37, 38]. However,

so far no trials have been reported in patients with carcinoma of the pancreas using somatostatin analogs.

Recent evidence indicates that growth factors play a role in pancreatic cancer. The fall in GH levels caused by somatostatin analogs [13, 16, 20, 21], could be important for the inhibition of pancreatic tumor growth. GH stimulates local production of insulin-like growth factor (IGF)-1 . IGF polypeptides, also called somatomedins, and various growth factors including epidermal growth factor (EGF), platelet- derived growth factor (PDGF), transforming growth factor (TGF) and others, appear to be involved in the proliferation of both normal and neoplastic cells or phenotypic transformation of cells [39-41]. PANC-1 and Mia PaCa-2 human pancreatic cancer cell lines have receptors for EGF [42, 43]. EGF stimulates the growth of Mia PaCa-2 pancreatic cancer cells in culture and may act as an autocrine growth factor [43]. EGF also augments pancreatic carcinogenesis induced by BOP [44]. Somatostatin reduces the levels of IGF-1 and EGF [16, 40, 41], and nullifies the cell replication in HeLa cells and growth of Mia PaCa-2 cells induced by EGF [43, 45]. In Mia PaCa-2 cancer cell lines, somatostatin reverses the stimulatory effect of EGF on the phosphorylation of the tyrosine kinase portion of the EGF receptor [46]. Some analogs of somatostatin, such as RC-160 and RC-121, are very activite in dephosphorylation of EGF receptors in the Mia PaCa-2 cell line. Somatostatin analogs might inhibit pancreatic cancers by suppressing the action or secretion of GI hormones and endogenous growth factors.

Sex steroids may also play a role in the growth of the normal and cancerous pancreas [9, 47-53]. The presence of specific receptors for estrogen and androgen in pancreatic cells indicates that sex hormones could influence neoplastic cell processes [9, 47-53]. Both androgen and estrogen receptors were detected in human pancreatic adenocarcinomas and cancer cell lines [9, 49-52]. That pancreatic adenocarcinomas might be sex steroid dependent is supported by the findings that testosterone stimulated the growth of xenografts of human pancreatic adenocarcinomas in nude mice whereas the antiandrogen cyproterone inhibited [49]. In human pancreatic cancers Greenway et al. detected aromatase and 5α-reductase, enzymes found only in sex steroid-dependent tissues [49].

Chronic administration of agonists of LHRH produces inhibition of the pituitary-gonadal axis manifested by decreased secretion of LH and FSH, and reduction in plasma levels of sex steroids [14]. The creation of a state of sex-hormone deprivation forms the main basis for oncological application of LH-RH agonists and can be used as an effective endocrine therapy for sex-hormone dependent cancers [14-16].

While repeated administration of LHRH agonists is required to reduce the levels of LH, FSH and sex steroids, similar effects can be obtained with a single administration of LHRH antagonists [14, 54, 55]. Thus both LHRH agonists and antagonists could be used for sex hormone deprivation in pancreatic cancer [11, 16].

EXPERIMENTAL STUDIES WITH HORMONAL THERAPY IN PANCREATIC CANCER

The experimental evidence is consistent with the view that the exocrine pancreatic carcinomas are sensitive to GI hormones, sex steroids and growth factors [13-17, 42-44, 46 49, 53] Inhibition of growth of pancreatic acinar and ductal carcinomas in animal models by analogues of hypothalamic hormones was first reported in 1984 [15]. The agonist [D-Trp^6]LHRH given daily or injected once a month in the form of controlled-release microcapsules, significantly decreased tumor weight and volume and suppressed serum testosterone levels. Chronic administration of some early somatostatin analogs also inhibited the growth of acinar pancreatic carcinomas in rats and of ductal cancers in hamsters [14, 15]. Modern somatostatin analogs such as RC-121 and RC-160 (D-Phe-Cys-Tyr-D-Trp-Lys-Val-Cys-Trp-NH$_2$) also inhibited the growth of transplanted or BOP-induced ductal pancreatic cancers in hamsters [16, 17]. Recently, Zalatnai and Schally [56] reported inhibition of tumor growth and evidence of histological regression of the BOP-induced pancreatic cancer in male hamsters after treatment with microcapsules of [D-Trp^6]LHRH or somatostatin analog RC-160. The combination of both peptides produced the best results in terms of prolongation of survival and histological regressive changes.

CLINICAL STUDIES WITH HORMONAL THERAPY

Clinical trials indicate that some patients with pancreatic cancer respond to the antiestrogen tamoxifen with prolongation of survival [9]. Since administration of LHRH agonists suppresses the levels of sex steroids, daily s.c. administration of [D-Trp^6]LHRH was tried clinically in patients with unresectable and histologically verified adenocarcinoma of the pancreas. This therapy led to clinical improvement and increase in survival in some patients [18]. One patient with stage IV disease lived for 16 months. In addition to subjective and objective improvement seen after 3 weeks of treatment, reduction in tumor mass and liver metastases was observed during laparotomy performed 11 months after the initiation of [D-Trp^6]LHRH [18].

CONCLUSIONS AND PROJECTIONS

Several mechanisms may be involved in the control of growth of pancreatic cancers. Administration of somatostatin analogs slows the growth of pancreatic tumors, possibly by inhibiting the secretion and/or action of GI hormones and growth factors. LHRH agonists decrease pancreatic tumor growth by eliminating the stimulatory effect of sex steroids. Combined administration of a somatostatin analog and an LHRH agonist, using long-acting delivery systems, might induce a greater inhibition of cancer of the pancreas than either alone.

ACKNOWLEDGEMENTS

The experimental work described in this paper was supported by
National Institutes of Health Grant CA 40077 and by the Medical
Research Service of the Veterans Administration.

REFERENCES

1.   Moossa, AR, Dawfon, PJ, Franklin, WA, Udekwu, AO and
Lavella-Jones, M (1986). Tumors of the pancreas. In: Moossa, AR,
Robson, MC and Schimpff, SC (eds.) "Comprehensive Textbook of
Oncology". p1105. (Baltimore; Williams and Wilkins).
2.   Connolly, MM, Dawson, PJ, Michelassi, F, Moossa, AR and
Lawenstein, F (1987). Survival in 1001 Patients with carcinoma of
the pancreas. Ann Surg, 206, 386
3.   Greenberger, JJ, Toskes, PP and Isselbacher, KJ (1987).
Diseases of the pancreas. In: Braunwald, E, Isselbacher, KJ,
Petersdorf, RG, Wilson, JD, Martin, JB and Fauci, AS (eds.)
"Harrison's Principles of Internal Medicine". 11th ed., p.1372.
(New York; McGraw-Hill Book Company).
4.   Journal Editorial (1986). Early diagnosis and screening for
pancreatic cancer. Lancet, 2, 785
6.   Douglass, HO Jr. (1987). Pancreatic Cancer: Nihilism is
Obsolete! Pancreas, 2, 230
7.   Blind, PJ and Dahlgren, ST (1987). Serum levels of the
carbohydrate antigen CA-50 in pancreatic disease. Acta Chir
Scand, 153, 45
8.   Smith, FP, Hoth, DF, Levin, B, Karlin, DA, Macdonald, JS,
Woolley, III PV and Schein, PS (1980). 5-Fluorouracil,
Adriamycin, and Mitomycin-C (FAM) chemotherapy for advanced
adenocarcinoma of the pancreas. Cancer, 46, 2014
9.   Theve, NO, Pousette, A and Carlstrom, K (1983).
Adenocarcinoma of the pancreas – a hormone sensitive tumor? A
preliminary report on nolvadex treatment. Clin Oncology, 9, 193
10.   Kalser, MH and Ellenberg, SS (1985). Pancreatic cancer:
adjuvant combined radiation and chemotherapy following curative
resection. Arch Surg, 120, 899
11.   Moertel, CG, Frytak, S, Hahn, RG, O'Connel, MJ, Reitemeier,
RJ, Rubin, J, Schutt, AJ, Weiland, LH, Childs, DS, Holbrook, MA,
Lavin, PT, Livstone, E, Spiro, H, Knowlton, A, Kalser, M, Barkin,
J, Lessner, H, Mann-Kaplan, R, Ramming, K, Douglas, Jr. HO,
Thomas, P, Nave, H, Bateman, J, Lokich, J, Brooks, J, Chaffey, J,
Corson, JM, Zamcheck, N and Novak, JW (1981). Therapy of locally
unresectable pancreatic carcinoma: a randomized comparison of high
dose (6000 rad) radiation alone, moderate dose radiation (4000
rad) + 5- fluorouracil and high dose radiation + 5-fluorouracil.
Cancer, 48, 1705
12.   Mallinson, CN, Rake, MO, Cocking, JB, Fox, CA, Cwynarski,
MT, Diffey, BL, Jackson, GA, Hanley, J and Wass, VJ (1980).
Chemotherapy in pancreatic cancer: results of a controlled,
prospective, randomised, multicentre trial. Brit Med J, 281, 1589
13.   Schally, AV, Cai, R-Z, Torres-Aleman, I, Redding, TW, Szoke,
B, Fu, D, Hierowski, MT, Colaluca, F and Konturek, S (1986).

Endocrine, gastrointestinal, and antitumor activity of
somatostatin analogues. In: Moody, TW (ed.) "Neural and Endocrine
Peptides and Receptors". p. 73. (New York; Plenum Press)
14. Schally, AV, Comaru-Schally, A-M and Redding, TW (1984).
Antitumor effects of analogs of hypothalamic hormones in
endocrine-dependent cancers. Proc Soc Exp Biol Med, 175, 259
15. Redding, TW and Schally, AV (1984). Inhibition of growth of
pancreatic carcinomas in animal models by analogs of hypothalamic
hormones. Proc Natl Acad Sci USA, 81, 248
16. Schally, AV, Redding, TW, Cai, R-Z, Paz, JI, Ben-David, M
and Comaru-Shally, A-M (1987). Somatostatin analogs in the
treatment of various experimental tumors. In: Klijn, JGM,
Paridaens, R and Foekens, JA (eds.) "Hormonal manipulation of
cancer: peptides, growth factors and new (anti) steroidal agents".
p.431. (New York; Raven Press).
17. Paz-Bouza, JI, Redding, TW and Schally, AV (1987).
Treatment of nitrosamine-induced pancreatic tumors in hamsters
with analogs of somatostatin and luteinizing hormone-releasing
hormone. Proc Natl Acad Sci USA, 84, 1112
18. Gonzalez-Barcena, D, Rangel-Garcia, NW, Perez-Sanches, PL,
Gutierrez-Dampiero, C, Garcia-Carrasco, F, Comaru-Schally, A-M and
Schally, AV (1986). Response to D-Trp-6-LH-RH in advanced
adenocarcinoma of pancreas. Lancet, 2, 154
19. Bauer, W, Briner, U, Doepfner, W, Haller, R, Huguenin, R,
Marbach, P, Petcher, TJ and Pless, J (1982). SMS-201-995: A very
potent and selective octapeptide analogue of somatostatin with
prolonged action. Life Sci, 31, 1133
20. Cai, RZ, Szoke, B, Lu, R, Fu, D, Redding, TW and Schally, AV
(1986). Synthesis and biological activity of highly potent
octapeptide analogs of somatostatin. Proc Natl Acad Sci USA, 83,
1896
21. Cai, RZ, Karashima, T, Gouth, J, Szoke, B, Olsen, D,
Schally, AV (1987). Superactive octapeptide somatostatin analogs
containing tryptophan residue in position 1. Proc. Natl Acad Sci,
USA, 84, 2502
22. Reichlin, S (1983). Somatostatin. New Engl J Med, 309, 1495
23. Konturek, SJ, Tasler, J, Cieszkowski, M, Coy, DH and
Schally, AV (1976). Effect of growth hormone release-inhibiting
hormone on gastric secretion, mucosal blood flow and serum
gastrin. Gastroenterology, 70, 737
24. Konturek, SJ, Tasler, J, Obtulowicz, W, Coy, DH and Schally,
AV (1976). Effect of growth hormone-release inhibiting hormone on
hormones stimulating exocrine pancreatic secretion. J Clin
Invest, 58, 1
25. Konturek, SJ, Cieszkowski, M, Bilski, J, Konturek, J,
Bielanski, W and Schally, AV (1985). Effects of cyclic
hexapeptide analog of somatostatin on pancreatic secretion in
dogs. Proc Soc Exp Biol Med, 178, 68
26. Konturek, SJ, Tasler, J, Krol, R, Dembinski, A, Coy, DH and
Schally, AV (1977). Effect of somatostatin analogs on gastric and
pancreatic secretion. Proc Soc Exp Biol Med, 155, 519
27. Schally, AV, Coy, DH and Meyers, CA (1978). Hypothalamic
regulatory hormones. Annu Rev Biochem, 47, 89

28. Mortimer, CH, Tunbridge, WMG, Carr, D, Yeomans, L, Lind, T, Coy, DH, Bloom, SR, Kastin, A, Mallinson, CN, Besser, GM, Schally, AV and Hall, R (1974). Effects of growth-hormone release-inhibiting hormone on circulating glucagon, insulin, and growth hormone in normal, diabetic, acromegalic, and hypo-pituitary patients. Lancet, 1, 697

29. Bloom, SR, Thorner, MO, Besser, GM, Hall, R, Gomez-Pan, A, Roy, VM, Russell, RCG, Coy, DH, Kastin, AJ and Schally, AV (1974). Inhibition of gastrin and gastric-acid secretion by growth-hormone release-inhibiting hormone. Lancet, 2, 1106

30. Johnson, LR (1981). Effects of gastrointestinal hormones on pancreatic growth. Cancer, 47, 1640

31. Dembinski, AB and Johnson, LR (1979). Growth of pancreas and gastrointestinal mucosa in antrectomized and gastrin-treated rats. Endocrinology, 105, 769

32. Dembinski, AB and Johnson, LR (1980). Stimulation of pancreatic growth by secretin, caerulein, and pentagastrin. Endocrinology, 106, 323

33. Sarfati, PD, Genik, P and Morisset, J (1985). Caerulein and secretin induced pancreatic growth: a possible control by endogenous pancreatic somatostatin. Regul Pept, 11, 263

34. Thompson, JC and Marx, M (1984). Gastrointestinal hormones. In: Ravitch, MM, Steichen, FM, Austen, WG, Scott, HW. Jr., Fonkaisrud, EW and Polk, HC, Jr. (eds.) "Current Problems in Surgery", vol. XXI, No.6, p.1-80. (Chicago; Year Book Medical Publishers, Inc.)

35. Townsend, CM, Franklin, RB, Watson, LC, Glass, EJ and Thompson, JC (1981). Stimulation of pancreatic cancer growth by caerulein and secretin. Surg Forum, 32, 228

36. Levison, DA (1979). Carcinoma of the pancreas. J Pathol, 129, 203

37. Vinik, AI, Tsai, S-T, Moattari, AR, Cheung, P, Eckhauser, FE and Cho, K (1986). Somatostatin analogue (SMS 201-995) in the management of gastroenteropancreatic tumors and diarrhea syndromes. Am J Med, 81, 23

38. Long, RG, Barnes, AJ, Adrian, TE, Mallinson, CM, Brown, MR, Vale, W, Rivier, JE, Christofides, ND and Bloom, SR (1979). Suppression of pancreatic endocrine tumor secretion by long-acting somatostatin analogue. Lancet, 2, 764

39. Goustin, AS, Leof, EB, Shipley, GD and Moses, HL (1986). Growth factors and cancer. Cancer Res, 46, 1015

40. Schally, AV and Redding TW (1987). Somatostatin analogs as adjuncts to agonists of luteinizing hormone-releasing hormone in the treatment of experimental prostate cancer. Proc Natl Acad Sci USA, 84, 7275

41. Setyono-Han, B, Henkelman, MS, Foekens, JA and Klijn, JGM (1987). Direct inhibitory effects of somatostatin (analogues) on the growth of human breast cancer cells. Cancer Res, 47, 1566

42. Korc, M and Magun, BE (1985). Recycling of epidermal growth factor in a human pancreatic carcinoma cell line. Proc Natl Acad Sci USA, 82, 6172

43. Liebow, C, Hierowski, M and DuSapin, K (1986). Hormonal control of pancreatic cancer growth. Pancreas, 1, 44

44.   Chester, JF, Gaissert, HA, Ross, JS and Malt, RA (1986). Pancreatic cancer in the Syrian hamster induced by N-Nitrobis (2-Oxopropyl)amine: cocarcinogenic effect of epidermal growth factor. Cancer Res, _46_, 2954

45.   Mascardo, RM and Sherline, P (1982). Somatostatin inhibits rapid centrosomal separation and cell proliferation induced by epidermal growth factor. Endocrinology, _111_, 1394

46.   Hierowski, MT, Liebow, C, Du Sapin, K and Schally, AV (1985). Stimulation by somatostatin of dephosphorylation of membrane proteins in pancreatic cancer MIA PaCa-2 cell line. FEBS Lett, _179_, 252

47.   Sandberg, A and Rosenthal, H (1979). Steroid receptors in exocrine glands: the pancreas and the prostate. J Steroid Biochem, _11_, 293

48.   Pousette, A (1976). Demonstration of an androgen receptor in rat pancreas. Biochem J, _157_, 229

49.   Greenway, B, Duke, D, Pym, B, Iqbal, MJ, Johnson, PJ and Williams, R (1982). The control of human pancreatic adenocarcinoma xenografts in nude mice by hormone therapy. Brit J Surg, _69_, 595

50.   Benz, C, Hollander, C and Miller, B (1986). Endocrine-responsive pancreatic carcinoma: steroid binding and cytotoxicity studies in human tumor cell lines. Cancer Res, _46_, 2276

51.   Corbishley, TP, Iqbal, MJ, Wilkinson, ML and Williams, R (1986). Androgen receptor in human normal and malignant pancreatic tissue and cell lines. Cancer, _57_, 1992

52.   Pousette, A, Carlstrom, K, Skoldefors, H, Wilking, N and Theve, NO (1982). Purification and partial characterization of a 17β-estradiol binding macro-molecule in the human pancreas. Cancer Res, _42_, 633

53.   Greenway, BA (1987). Carcinoma of the exocrine pancreas: sex hormone responsive tumour? Brit J Surg, _74_, 441

54.   Schally, AV (1983). Current status of antagonistic analogs of LH-RH as a contraceptive method in the female. Res Front Fertil Reg, _2_, 1

55.   Debeljuk, L and Schally, AV (1986). Antifertility effects of a potent LH-RH antagonist in male and female rats. Int J Fertil, _31_, 284

56.   Zalatnai, A and Schally, AV (1988). Responsiveness of the hamster pancreatic cancer to treatment with microcapsules of [D-Trp[6]]LHRH and somatostatin analog RC-160: histological evidence of improvement. Int J Pancreatol, in press

20
AN FSH PRODUCING TUMOR: RESPONSE TO GnRH ANALOGUE

M. BEREZIN, H. HALKIN and **B. LUNENFELD**
Institute of Endocrinology and Department A of Internal Medicine,
The Chaim Sheba Medical Center, Tel Hashomer 52621, Israel, and
Tel Aviv University, Sackler School of Medicine, Tel Aviv, Israel

INTRODUCTION

Gonadotropin-producing pituitary adenomas are rare. Only about 25 such patients have been reported [1]. In 1984 we described a very aggressive isolated FSH producing pituitary tumor in a 32 year old fertile man with normal sperm [2]. Most of the reported patients were men with histories of primary hypogonadism and secondary elevation of FSH levels [1]. In four patients a combination of increased levels of FSH and LH were detected [1,3-5]. Isolated elevated LH secretion was reported in two patients [6,7]. The simultaneous hypersecretion of TSH and FSH and the excessive production of an abnormal form of FSH has also recently been described [8,9]. Most patients presented with macroadenoma and visual field defects and were treated by irradiation and/or pituitary adenomectomy [1]. We here report on treatment of an FSH producing tumor with a GnRH analogue.

Effect of a GnRH Agonist

After repeated surgery and external irradiation therapy the tumor size in our patient remained unchanged (Fig. 1). The patient was blind and the plasma FSH level was highly elevated (240 mIU/ml).
The FSH secretion increased following GnRH administration (Fig. 2), paradoxically increased after TRH administration (Table 1) and was decreased following a single dose of 5 mg bromocriptine (Table 2).

Table 1. Hormonal response to i.v. administration of 200 µg TRH

Hormone	Basal	Maximal
FSH (mIU/ml)	243	321
LH (mIU/ml)	3.5	7
TSH (mIU/ml)	5.1	11
hPRL (ng/ml)	18	24.7

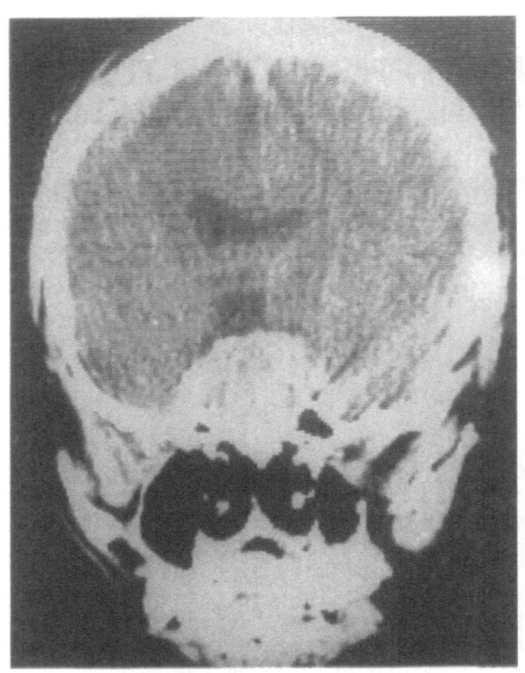

FIGURE 1   Coronal scan revealed a large sella mass with
significant suprasellar extension

Table 2.   FSH, LH, and PRL responses to a single dose of 5 mg
bromocriptine

Time (min)	LH (mIU/ml)	FSH (mIU/ml)	hPRL (ng/ml)
0	2.3	137	12.7
60	1.5	141.8	8.6
120	<1.0	123.4	4.4
180	<1.0	82.8	3.6
240	<1.0	79.4	3.5
300	<1.0	64.4	2.9

Since neither sex steroids nor neurotransmitters were
capable of inhibiting FSH production or shrinking the tumor mass
and no GnRH agonists were available in 1981, a therapeutic trial
with bromocriptine was made.   FSH levels decreased from 240 mIU/ml
to 40 mIU/ml and remained on this level for 6 years (Fig. 3).
However, no shrinkage of the tumor mass was observed.

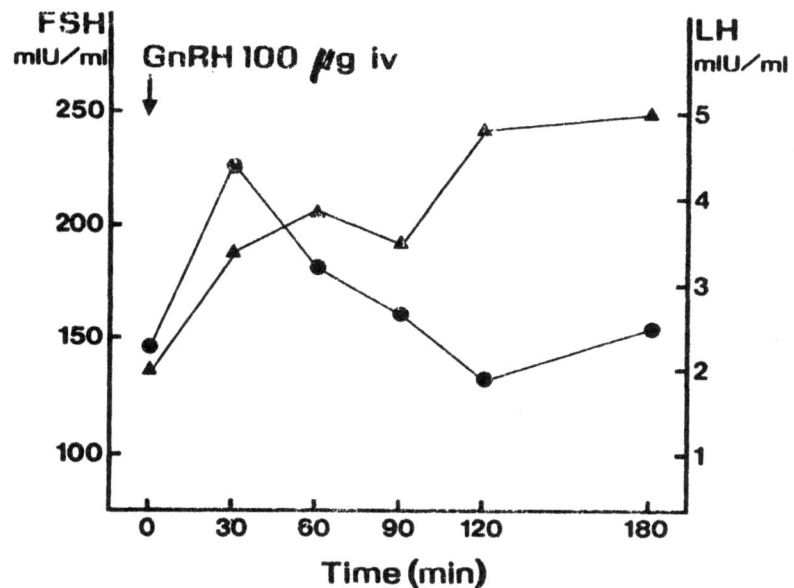

FIGURE 2 Responses of FSH (▲——▲) and LH (●——●) to iv
injection of 100 µg GnRH, 1 month after irradiation
treatment.

With the availability of GnRH agonist and the fact that the
tumor was responsive to native GnRH an attempt was made to treat
the patient with Decapeptil in a long acting formulation.
Bromocriptine treatment was stopped and two weeks thereafter a
GnRH test was performed to reconfirm the response of the tumor to
GnRH.

The base level of 40 mIU/ml of FSH observed during
bromocriptine treatment increased to 98.5 mIU/ml after two weeks
following cessation of bromocriptine therapy. 100 µg of native
GnRH caused an FSH increase to 164 mIU/ml showing a positive
response to GnRH (Table 3).

Table 3. GnRH test (100 mcg im) (1987)

Time	FSH mIU/ml	LH mIU/ml	Testosterone ng/ml	PRL ng/ml
0	98.5	17.0	8.4	22.7
+15'	97.5	21.0	4.8	27.5
+30'	142.5	23.5	5.3	22.2
+60'	164.5	31.0	6.4	22.4

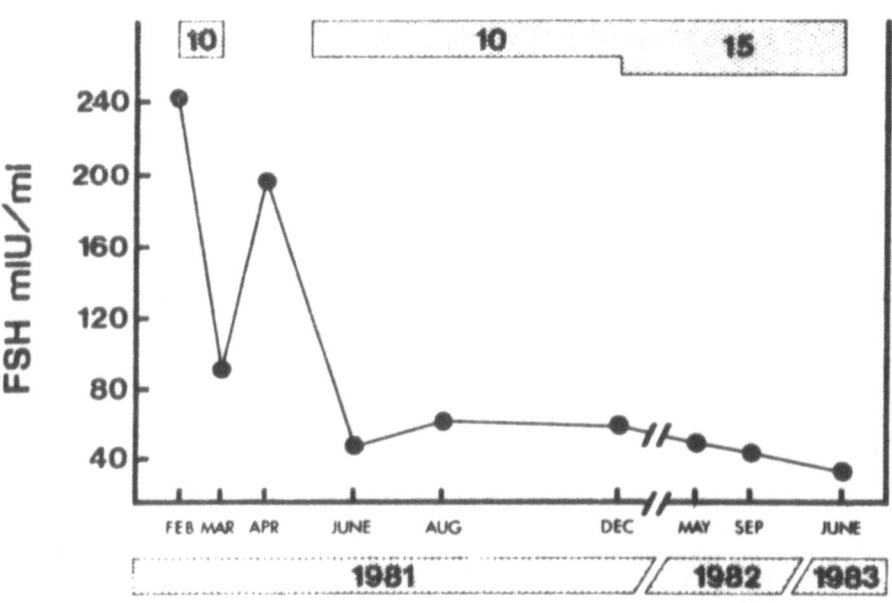

FIGURE 3 FSH leves during a 28-month period of treatment with bromocriptine. Note the rapid decrease of FSH after 3 weeks of bromocriptine treatment (10 mg/day), its rise again after stopping treatment, and the sustained low levels during continuous treatment.

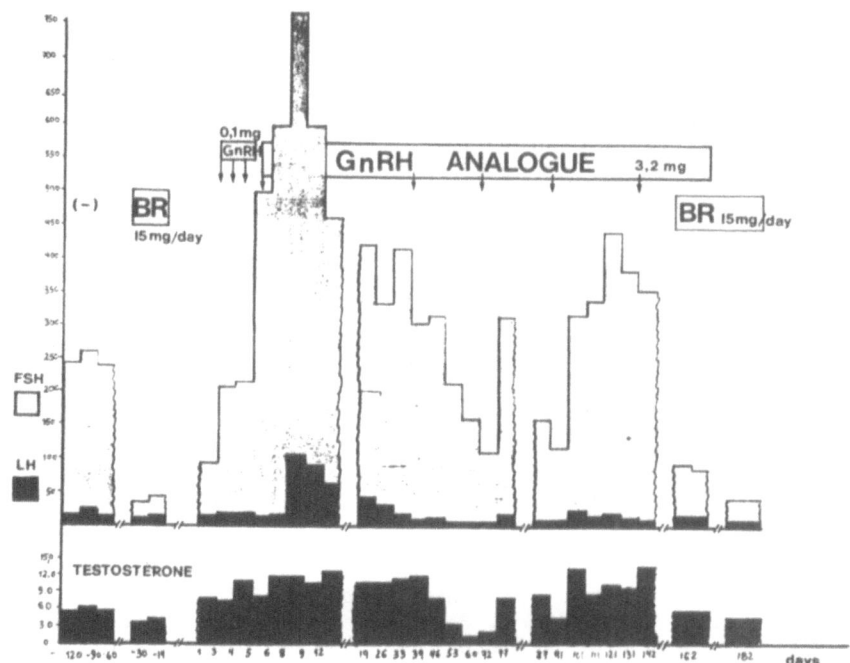

FIGURE 4 FSH, LH and testosterone during the treatment with
Decapeptil and Bromocriptine.

An initial administration of 100 mcg of Decapeptil for 3
consecutive days stimulated FSH secretion to 220 mIU/ml.
Concomitantly an increase of LH and testosterone was observed.

Since the treatment was well tolerated by the patient and
there was an absence of side effects such as headache, nausea or
other signs of increase of intracranial pressure, we continued the
treatment with high dosage of GnRH analogue - 3.2 mg every
28-30 days (Fig. 4).

Within 3 days the FSH level rose to 760 mIU/ml.
Concomitantly LH and testosterone increased. Thereafter a gradual
decline of FSH and LH was noted. Following the second injection,
instead of the stimulatory effect on FSH and LH, both gonadotropic
hormones continued to decrease. After the third injection, on
day 72, FSH increased and immunoreactive LH remained at
pretreatment basal levels, whereas testosterone was 40% higher
than prior to treatment.

Both the fourth and the fifth injections evoked an initial
stimulatory effect on FSH production. Since FSH continued to

fluctuate between 325-340 mIU/ml, bromocriptine treatment was reinstated on day 142, while the GnRH analogue injections were continued. The FSH level dropped to 97 mIU/ml, which was however significantly higher than during bromocriptine treatment alone.

Since the patient developed a painful bilateral gynecomastia, we stopped the GnRH analogue treatment and continued bromocriptine alone. This resulted in further reduction of FSH levels without change in LH and testosterone levels, similar to the first bromocriptine treatment period.

CONCLUSIONS

It can be concluded that secretion of FSH in this isolated FSH producing tumor could be stimulated by native GnRH and its analogue, and also paradoxically by TRH. It could be suppressed by prolonged GnRH analogue administration, but bromocriptine was capable of significantly suppressing FSH levels.

This demonstrates the autonomous and unspecific nature of this isolated FSH producing tumor.

REFERENCES

1.   Nicolis, GL, Modhi, G, and Gabrilove, JL (1982). Gonadotropin producing pituitary adenomas. A case report and review of the literature. Mt Sinai J Med, 49, 297
2.   Berezin, M, Olchovsky, D, Pines, A, Tadmor, R and Lunenfeld, B (1984). Reduction of follicle - stimulating hormone (FSH) - secretion in FSH - producing pituitary adenoma by bromocriptine. J Clin Endocrinol Metab, 59, 1220
3.   Demura, R, Kuba, O, Demura, H, and Shizume, K (1977). FSH and LH secreting pituitary adenoma. J Clin Endocrinol Metab, 45, 653
4.   Kovacs, K, Horwath, E, Rewcastle, NB and Ezrin, C (1980). Gonadotroph cell adenoma of the pituitary in a woman with longstanding hypogonadism. Arch Gynecol, 229, 57
5.   Snyder, PJ, and Sterling FH (1976). Hypersecretion of LH and FSH by pituitary adenoma. J Clin Endocrinol Metab, 2, 554
6.   Burke, CW, and Marshall, JC (1971). Ovarian failure with probable pituitary tumor. Proc Roy Soc Lond (Biol), 64, 1066
7.   Peterson, RE, Kourides, IA, Horwith, M. Vaughan, ED, Saxen, BB and Fraser, AR (1981). LH secreting pituitary tumor and subunit: positive feedback of estrogen. J Clin Endocrinol Metab, 54, 692
8.   Koide, Y, Kugai, N, Kimura, S, Fujita, T, Kameya, T, Azukizawa, M, Ogata, E, Tomono, Y and Yamashita, K (1982). A case of pituitary adenoma with possible simultaneous secretion of thyrotropin and follicle - stimulating hormone. J Clin Endocrinol Metab, 54, 397
9.   Wide, L, and Lundberg, PO (1981). Hypersecretion of an abnormal form of follicle stimulating hormone associated with suppressed luteinizing hormone secretion in a woman with a pituitary adenoma. J Clin Endocrinol Metab, 53, 923

INDEX

217

218

221

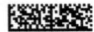